Life without Disease

UNIVERSITY OF CALIFORNIA PRESS

Life without Disease

THE PURSUIT OF MEDICAL UTOPIA

WILLIAM B. SCHWARTZ, M.D.

BERKELEY   LOS ANGELES   LONDON

University of California Press
Berkeley and Los Angeles, California

University of California Press, Ltd.
London, England

Library of Congress Cataloging-in-
Publication Data

Schwartz, William B., 1922–
    Life without disease : the pursuit of
medical utopia / William B. Schwartz.
        p.   cm.
    Includes bibliographic references
and index.
        ISBN 0–520–21467–6 (alk. paper)
        1. Medical innovations—social as-
pects.   2. Medical technology—social
aspects.   3. Managed care plans (Medical care)   I. Title.   RA418.5.M4S39   1998
    610—dc 21   97–41639

Printed in the United States of America
9 8 7 6 5 4 3 2 1

To my precious wife, Tressa, and in memory of my son Kenneth

Contents

Preface

Millions of Americans find themselves by turns intrigued, mystified, frustrated, and downright scared by the constantly changing face of medical care in the 1990s. Scarcely a day goes by without major news stories on a medical breakthrough or on the impending insolvency of Medicare and the threat of rationing by health care providers. Even as the public is offered an endless string of medical success stories, they are reminded that health care insurers have unceremoniously thrown new mothers out of the hospital the day after delivery. Policymakers are one day touting managed care as the solution to spiraling health care costs and the next day beating the drum to outlaw measures used by managed care plans to save money. Competing hospital networks carry on confusing advertising wars that make the long distance phone companies look like duffers, and every week seems to bring a new buyout or merger between health care conglomerates. A welter of medical, ethical, economic, political, and legal issues swirl around these developments, and it is small wonder that many Americans wonder whether the country is headed toward a medical utopia or a medical meltdown.

This book is my attempt to provide a framework for understanding how the pieces of this complex puzzle fit together. To understand this critical moment in the U.S. health care system, it is necessary to appreciate both how we have arrived at the current state of affairs and where we may be headed in the coming decades. For this reason, the book tells its story chronologically, beginning with the medical research boom of the 1950s and ending in 2050. The story is also of necessity a multidisciplinary one, embracing economics, public policy, ethics, medical research, and clinical care. Only by viewing these components in relation to one another is it possible to bring order out of the jumble of news flashes, editorial pronouncements, legislative edicts, and corporate PR with which we are all bombarded.

I bring to this task my experience as a physician-in-chief of a major teaching hospital who took a midcareer detour from clinical medicine into the field of health care economics and public policy. My experience as a clinician has made me an unashamed enthusiast for the triumphs of medical progress that have occurred since the beginning of my professional career some decades ago, and an optimist about the potential for even more dramatic successes in the decades ahead. However, in a series of op-ed pieces for the *New York Times*, the *Washington Post*, and the *Wall Street Journal*, and articles published in the *Journal of the American Medical Association* and the *New England Journal of Medicine*, I have espoused the unpopular idea that the rapid rise in health care costs resulting from our medical successes cannot be controlled without the acceptance of painful but necessary limits on the availability of certain expensive treatments to some or all patients. The recent transformation of the U.S. health care system into one dominated by managed care organizations has only brought into sharper focus the inevitable clash between cost containment efforts and the view of medical care as an unlimited entitlement.

In writing this book during the past five years, I have reached out to many friends and colleagues for advice and assistance. Three individuals in particular have made invaluable contributions:

David Morse, Associate Director of the Norris Medical Library at the University of Southern California, who served throughout this project as editor, critic, and sounding board, and without whose assistance the book could not have reached the level of clarity it has; Daniel Mendelson, vice president of the Lewin Group in Fairfax, Virginia, who generously shared his considerable expertise on matters of health policy and made available the efficient fact-finding resources of the Lewin Group; and my wife, Tressa Miller, who at several stages of this project read the entire manuscript and helped me to make the story more understandable, more humane, and more relevant to the concerns of the general reader. My wife also withstood for three years the erratic and preoccupied behavior of a struggling author with singular forbearance and generosity of spirit, for which I am forever in her debt.

Among the many colleagues at the University of Southern California who provided helpful advice are: Michael Bolger, David Faxon, Donald Feinstein, Eva Henriksen, Laurence Kedes, Michael Kline, Aruna Patil, Arnold Platzker, Kumar Rajamani, and Andrew Stoltz. I have also called upon the assistance of colleagues from my years at the Tufts University School of Medicine, including Marshall Kaplan, Barry Fanburg, Herbert Levine, Nicolaos Madias, and Stephen Pauker.

A further group of individuals who generously shared their expertise are Kurt Isselbacher, Toshihiro Shiodo, and Sheridan Kassirer at the Massachusetts General Hospital/Brigham and Women's Hospital; Donald Schon at the Massachusetts Institute of Technology; Barry Barish at the California Institute of Technology; Belding Scribner at the University of Washington School of Medicine; Charles van Ypersele at the University of Louvain; Daniel Ortiz at the University of Virginia; Andrew Dreyfus of the Massachusetts Hospital Association; and Kellie Mitra and Jennifer Shapiro, Daniel Mendelson's assistants at the Lewin Group.

Several individuals reviewed the entire manuscript and provided valuable criticisms: Edward Crandall, David Goldstein, and Steven Ryan at the University of Southern California; and Joseph Miller, a Los Angeles–based attorney. Henry Aaron of the Brookings Institution, who has over many years been a stimulating and valued colleague, provided a particularly thoughtful review of the chapters on health economics.

I am indebted to Provost Sol Gittelman of Tufts University, whose unflagging encouragement and enthusiasm were so important to me during my years of research at Tufts. I also want to express my deep appreciation to Richard Tannen, former chairman of the University of Southern California Department of Medicine, who invited me to join the faculty at USC.

Funding support provided by the University of Southern California School of Medicine, the Pacific Center for Health Policy and Ethics, and the Distinguished Physician Program of the Department of Veterans Affairs gave me time to undertake the extended research and writing that this book has required. The David and Sylvia Weisz Foundation also provided financial support in the preliminary phases of my research.

To all of these individuals and organizations I again offer my heartfelt thanks.

William B. Schwartz, M.D.
Department of Medicine
University of Southern California School of Medicine

Humankind's age-old attempt to stave off disease has been influenced not only by the progress of science but also by a changing vision of what science can achieve. That vision may now be due for a major transformation as our exploding knowledge of the genetic mechanisms of disease begins to make plausible the once impossible dream of a largely disease-free existence. The fulfillment of the dream is of course dependent on a host of future developments that cannot be predicted accurately, but at least the possibility of a broad-based victory over disease and a dramatic increase in the human lifespan in the not too remote future must now be taken seriously. This reimagining of our medical future seems all the more important in light of growing scientific evidence that the aging process itself may be subject to medical intervention. The myriad social and economic repercussions likely to result from these scientific victories make it prudent to begin envisioning the benefits as well as the attendant problems of the medical utopia that may be on the horizon.

The dream of a human existence freed from the scourges of disease and old age is probably as old as the human imagination itself, but it was the great Enlightenment thinkers of the seventeenth and eighteenth centuries who first suggested that the dream might have a scientific basis. The philosopher René Descartes wrote, for instance, that "we might be free of an infinity of maladies both of body and mind, and even of the infirmities of old age, if we had sufficient knowledge of their causes and remedies."[1] A century later Benjamin Franklin echoed the scientific euphoria of the age in forecasting the day when "all diseases may by sure means be prevented or cured, not excepting that of old age, and our lives lengthened at pleasure even beyond the antediluvian standard."[2]

However, in the years that followed, such dreams faded as scientists began to appreciate the complexity and elusiveness of human health. Even the prospect of dependable and sustained progress against disease—let alone the achievement of a medical utopia—emerged only after World War II, fueled by the explosive growth of the U.S. National Institutes of Health. A succession of major medical advances quickly proved the efficacy of government-supported medical research. The modern era of medical discovery—and the story of this book—gets its start in these years. Not coincidentally, these years also witnessed the discovery of the structure of DNA, by which the seeds were planted for a revival of medicine's utopian aspirations through the tools of cellular genetics.

The period covered by this book is roughly the hundred-year span—of which we are now at the midpoint—beginning with the birth of the modern health care industry in the 1950s and ending in the year 2050, when many of today's adults will still be living, and when it seems conceivable that most of today's debilitating and fatal diseases will be preventable or curable. The first half-century of this period has been characterized by extraordinary advances in the way medicine can diagnose and repair the ravages of disease—from hip replacement and angioplasty to completely new diagnostic tools like magnetic resonance imaging (MRI) and computed tomography (CT). Significantly, however, few of these advances have offered a basis for utopian aspiration, focused as they have been on battling the effects rather than the root causes of disease.

In the half-century to come, the emerging field of molecular medicine, which exploits the science of molecular biology and genetics to attack disease processes at their subcellular origins, promises to usher in a new era of vastly more effective care. Dr. Alfred Gilman, a 1996 Nobel Laureate, described one aspect of the new era this way: "In perhaps 50 years every molecule in the human body will be known. You'll be able to design a drug that works only on the molecule you want and on no other molecule in the body."[3] This new medicine, instead of treating the consequences of disease as in the past, will concentrate on the genetic causes of disease, on preventive measures for patients with genetic predisposition to disease, and on new ways to interrupt the pathways that lead from genes to diseases.

Given the immense therapeutic potential of molecular interventions, it does not seem at all unlikely that the child born at the close of this amazing hundred-year period could enjoy a life expectancy of 130 years or more and be free of the major chronic illnesses that now plague the aging. That is the utopian vision for medicine that now, for the first time, appears to have a scientific foundation.

The critical question is at what price—economically, politically, and ethically—that vision will be realized. As we will see, there is already ample evidence that the current turmoil in the U.S. health care system derives in no small part from its growing success in understanding and mastering disease.

Part One

Halfway to Utopia

1950 to 2000

1

The Birth and Growth
of Big Medicine

As the United States emerged triumphant from World War II, scientists and government leaders came to a conclusion that was to have momentous implications. Looking at the obvious success of research efforts like the Manhattan Project, they reasoned that similarly aggressive government support of medical research could yield equally dramatic results. These were not utopian dreamers but simply pragmatists who understood how much could be accomplished by research scientists supported by a generously funded and well-coordinated government program. There is no evidence that they anticipated the scale of either the costs or the success of the technological revolution they were about to unleash on the American health care system. But they did understand that medical progress costs money, and they believed that the American people were ready to harness some of the nation's growing economic muscle in the fight against disease.

One such believer was Mary Lasker, a wealthy and successful businesswoman, who, along with her equally wealthy and determined husband, Albert, helped weld together a coalition of public and private leaders dedicated to putting medical research funding on the national political agenda. The Laskers were able to exploit their friendships with influential physicians like Sidney Farber and

Michael Debakey, and with powerful politicians like Senators Lister Hill of Alabama and Claude Pepper of Florida, to further their cause. One of Mary Lasker's first accomplishments was to transform the American Cancer Society from a relatively unimportant support organization into a major source of money for medical research. She soon realized, however, that only the government sector could hope to amass the sums necessary to tackle such intractable medical challenges as cancer, heart disease, and mental illness. She therefore turned her forceful will, her unrivaled social connections, and her deep pockets toward the political arena, where she set a new standard for concerted and effective congressional lobbying. She contributed heavily to election campaigns, befriended presidents, charmed the press, and built a network of like-minded movers and shakers, memorably described by Elizabeth Drew in an *Atlantic Monthly* article titled "The Health Syndicate: Washington's Noble Conspirators."[1] As a direct result of these efforts, the National Institutes of Health (NIH) began its rise from a small agency with a budget of $26 million in 1948 to the Goliath it is today, with an estimated 1997 budget of $12.4 billion.[2]

Today we take for granted the steady stream of medical discoveries issuing from the nation's medical schools and research laboratories, but this phenomenon is heavily dependent on a system of government-funded research invented less than fifty years ago. At the time, no one could have guessed that the new commitment to medical research might sow the seeds not only of a revolution in health care but also of a seemingly irresistible growth in overall health care expenditures.

In 1950 costs of health care were remarkably low, because, for a large percentage of patients, doctors really couldn't do much. People spent relatively little on health care (only 4.4 percent of gross domestic product) and got what they paid for—very few useful diagnostic tests or effective treatments.[3] A basic physical examination, simple blood tests, and diagnostic X-rays of the chest, bowel, and bone could reveal a few treatable diseases, but many other diseases that are today well controlled by drugs led in those days to complete incapacitation. Patients with severe congestive heart failure spent their days in padded chairs designed to keep the edema from settling in their lungs. Patients with uncontrollable angina pectoris were effectively disabled, incapable of walking more than a few yards before being brought up short by severe chest pain. Those suffering from malignant hypertension were at the mercy of severe headaches, loss of vision, and eventual kidney failure or stroke. In the absence of effective diagnostic methods for many abdominal diseases, exploratory surgery was the less than satisfactory alternative.

Hospital care was almost untouched by technology. Pulmonary problems were treated with oxygen tents, but ventilators to improve oxygen and carbon dioxide exchange more effectively were not available. Intensive care units were unheard of. Very ill patients who could afford it hired private-duty nurses to provide personal hospital care, but these nurses had almost no equipment to work with and little specialized training.

The world of medicine changed quickly, however, once the federal government began to bankroll the nation's biomedical research effort. By 1950, Congress had provided the National Institutes of Health with a splendid new facility in Bethesda, along with a burgeoning annual budget to support research at the NIH itself and at medical schools throughout the country. The result between 1950 and 1970 was a dramatic increase in the pace of medical discovery. Treatments were developed for hitherto intractable illnesses such as hypertension, kidney failure, inflammatory bowel disease, childhood leukemia, and many infections. Medical care and its associated costs were transfigured by the introduction of the first high-technology treatment modalities, such as intensive care units, kidney transplantation, retinal surgery, and replacement of damaged heart valves.

CHRONIC DIALYSIS:
HARBINGER OF THE MEDICAL TECHNOLOGY BOOM

One of the most dramatic advances of the postwar decades was the use of the artificial kidney for the treatment of chronic kidney failure. This technology, highly effective but extremely expensive, was the first real budget-buster in the medical arsenal and, as such, the forerunner of the explosion of high-priced technologies that have created the current crisis in health care costs. The story of the beginnings of chronic kidney dialysis, all but forgotten after 45 years, still offers lessons on how decisions about patient care are reached when a medical technology outstrips the available resources.

Chronic progressive renal failure is a devastating and invariably fatal disorder. When toxic waste products are not fully excreted by the kidneys, they accumulate in the blood and cause a variety of symptoms such as loss of appetite, nausea, vomiting, and general weakness. In the last stages of kidney failure, the buildup of waste products causes severe itching, debilitation, mental confusion, and convulsions. As a nephrologist in the 1950s, before the introduction of chronic dialysis, I was frustrated and saddened as I watched patients deteriorate in such a terrible way. Sympathy with their plight and concern for their comfort were almost all that I or any physician could offer them. Transplantation of a healthy kidney, except between identical twins, was still a distant dream because of the unsolved problems of rejection of foreign tissue.

The first artificial kidney, developed in the 1940s, was practical for use in patients with short-term and reversible acute kidney failure, but not for the long-term treatment of chronic kidney failure. The device is basically a large cylinder filled with a solution into which the toxic blood products can diffuse and be eliminated. A catheter is placed in an artery and attached to tubing that leads blood through the "washing machine" and then returns the cleansed blood to the body through another catheter inserted in a vein. In the 1940s and 1950s, the device could be used only in acute cases because the catheters began to cause problems after about a week; infection of the catheterized vessels or a blood clot at the catheter site often barred further treatment.

No one except Dr. Belding Scribner of Seattle ever believed that a catheter might be designed that could be left in place for a prolonged period and would therefore allow treatment for months or years of chronic kidney failure. But all the skeptics (including myself) were wrong. In the early 1960s, Scribner designed a catheter that could be used for an extended period. He then showed that with repeated dialysis, even patients with long-term kidney failure could enjoy a reasonably comfortable life. Almost immediately patients flocked to Seattle seeking treatment in Scribner's facility and overwhelmed its available beds and machines. Grant support for the effort was modest, and medical insurance would not cover the procedure, so only patients who could pay the entire cost, about $30,000 a year, were accepted. Even this expense, however, did not deter a large pool of patients from applying for treatment.

Given the limited facilities, some process for choosing among the hundreds of desperate and dying patients seeking treatment had to be devised. After an advisory committee of physicians weeded out the candidates who were least promising from a strictly medical point of view, a second committee of ordinary citizens from the community was given the task of deciding which of the remaining patients should be saved. This "life or death" committee operated in a shroud of secrecy. Its deliberations were never public, and its membership was unknown to those whose lives it held in the balance. An early television program on the subject showed chilling clips of a committee meeting in session, with each member's face obscured. The committee's deliberations have been described this way.

Formal criteria for decision-making were not actually used by the lay committee. But in making its decisions, it considered the follow-

ing: the ability of a housewife from eastern Washington to move to
Seattle; the relative importance of saving a parent with two children
compared to one with six; the prospect for rehabilitation and return
to work; the potential of "service to society" based on education;
the candidate's "character and moral strength" based on church
membership; and the probable opportunity of the surviving spouse
to remarry.[4]

The selection process represented the first explicit rationing of
high-tech health care in the United States. Not unexpectedly, the
American public and its elected representatives reacted with dismay
at the prospect of people dying for no reason other than insufficient
facilities and money. After a modest expansion of dialysis programs, most notably in the Veterans Administration hospitals, the
federal government was coaxed into full funding of dialysis in the
mid-1960s, largely because of support by Representative Wilbur
Mills, the extremely powerful chair of the House of Representatives
Ways and Means Committee. At the behest of several well-known
nephrologists, Mills allowed a "live" dialysis to be carried out before his committee.[5] (The proposed demonstration was viewed
with trepidation by many other nephrologists, who felt that a ca-
tastrophe could occur during the procedure and discredit the entire
dialysis program for the foreseeable future.)

On November 4, 1971, an artificial kidney was wheeled into a
congressional hearing room, and a patient was dialyzed in the presence of a group of awed representatives. As some had feared, a
significant complication did occur in the course of the procedure—the onset of a serious cardiac arrhythmia—and the
procedure had to be terminated before it was completed. The representatives, however, were unaware of the problem, and it is generally agreed that this demonstration was a key factor in the
congressional vote to fund chronic dialysis treatments. Who, after
all, could resist the urge to alleviate the plight of this man and his
fellow sufferers—particularly if the price was manageable? An im-

portant factor in the congressional decision to fund dialysis was the experts' projection that costs would be relatively modest.

Support for the effort also came from the Senate side. One strong advocate was Washington Senator Henry "Scoop" Jackson, who had a relative on dialysis in Seattle. Senator Jackson felt that it was "a great tragedy, in a nation as affluent as ours, that we have to consciously make a decision all over America as to the people who will live and the people who will die." Senator Lawton Chiles of Florida, honorary chair of the Florida Kidney Foundation, was equally disturbed that "in this country with so much affluence . . . there are people who will die this year merely because we do not have enough of these machines and do not have enough dollars, so that we have to make the choice of who will live and who will die, when we already know we have a good treatment that can succeed and keep these people alive while we are working out other improvements in transplants, finding cures, and everything else necessary. This should not happen in this country."[6]

Shortly thereafter, in 1972, a new provision was added to the Social Security Act entitling every patient, rich or poor, to free dialysis and all care related to it. The benefits to patients in kidney failure have been enormous. Some 250,000 Americans now have their lives sustained by some form of dialysis. The costs have also proved to be enormous, soaring to some $8 billion in 1994 for the treatment of patients in the End Stage Renal Disease Program.[7] In funding dialysis, Congress ushered in an era in which high technology was to become both a medical blessing and a financial curse. Over the following decades, imaginative scientists, funded generously by the NIH, produced a string of similarly useful and expensive new technologies: transplantation of heart, liver, and lung, new imaging techniques, hip and other joint replacement, coronary bypass grafts, and cardiac pacemakers. The burden of paying for these other new technologies, however, remained largely with patients and their insurers.

U.S. MEDICINE COMES OF AGE

Bringing medical advances to the patient required far more than new tests and treatments. More sophisticated and specialized care demanded more and better-trained doctors, more hospitals, and, above all, more money. No master plan existed for reallocating national resources to the health care sector, but an exceptional conjunction of social and political forces allowed all the pieces to fall into place by the mid-1960s. First, federal legislation in the 1940s stimulated large increases in the number of hospital beds. Subsequent federal actions encouraged growth in the number of medical schools and size of medical classes, thus increasing the supply of physicians. Paying for new care was facilitated by the rapid spread of employer-paid health insurance and by the advent of Medicare and Medicaid in 1965—now even the previously underserved elderly and disabled, as well as many of the poor, gained access to care.

By 1970, a revolution in health insurance had occurred, with some 80 percent of all Americans insured, and with benefits covering, on average, 50 percent of medical bills.[8] This increase in coverage led to a change in the public's attitude toward health services. The newly insured no longer had any incentive to moderate their demands on the health care system but instead demanded the best that the system could offer. And physicians, for their part, felt free to err routinely on the side of overtreating, in some instances to enhance their own income and in others to protect themselves against the perceived threat of malpractice suits (practicing so-called "defensive" medicine).

Insulated from the brunt of the full costs of health care, patients and physicians alike became less concerned with medical expenses, and normal market forces that had previously acted as a brake on costs began to weaken. Expenditures on health care grew by 1970 to 7.4 percent of the gross domestic product—a substantial figure, but one that at first evoked no great concern on the part of policymakers or the public.[9] That rise, however, augured a trend that would, two decades later, bring the rate of increase in costs to the top tier of national concerns. In the meantime, with generous research support from the NIH continuing to flow and health insurance making top-flight medicine available even to patients of modest means, the scene was set for a new age of medical miracles and soaring costs.

THE QUIET REVOLUTION OF MOLECULAR BIOLOGY

Eclipsed by the highly visible progress in clinical medicine was another scientific revolution. In the nation's genetic research laboratories, the foundations were beingeing laid for a radical transformation in biomedical science. In the first half of this century, scientists struggled to solve the fundamental mystery of how an individual's genes are stored in cells and passed on to new cells as they are formed. The work culminated in the 1940s with the conclusion that the vehicle that carried the crucial genetic information was deoxyribonucleic acid (DNA). During the early 1950s, scientists avidly pursued the structure of DNA, with the hope of understanding how genetic information was encoded and reproduced. Francis Crick and James Watson made the groundbreaking discovery that the DNA molecule is configured as a double helix—a design that allows genes to be copied accurately from one cell to another. These insights led, in turn, to an explosion of research on how specific genes are translated into the unique structural and biochemical features of individuals, including their susceptibility to disease.

This work in molecular biology continues to gain momentum. In our century perhaps only the discoveries of quantum mechanics and the introduction of psychoanalytic thought have come close to rivaling the sweeping impact of molecular biology, which has revolutionized our understanding of life itself. But in the 1950s and 1960s, almost no one outside the scientific community appreciated how radically clinical care might eventually be changed by genetic approaches to disease.

TECHNOLOGY BLOOMS AND THE COST CRISIS LOOMS: 1975–2000

In recent decades, money for medical research has continued to flow in an ever wider stream from the federal government. Regardless of which political party held a majority, Congress has treated medical research as a favored child, with appropriations often exceeding the budget requests of the President. Rapid medical advances have been assimilated into a health care system in which well-funded hospitals, an abundance of doctors, and a thriving health insurance industry assured a friendly reception. As a result, medical advances have flourished. When patients now complain about the escalating costs of care, they generally forget that many of the therapies available to them were unimaginable just a few years ago: many of today's most familiar tools of medical care had their debut after 1975.

The introduction of noninvasive techniques, in particular, had a major effect on medical practice, effecting a shift from traumatic and risky surgical procedures to approaches such as computed tomography scanning, ultrasound, and magnetic resonance imaging. No longer was it necessary to drill through the skull in search of tumors, aneurysms, or blood clots or to open up the abdomen to diagnose unexplained abdominal pain. The traumatic effects of abdominal surgery, such as gall bladder removal, were minimized with laparoscopy—the use of miniaturized surgical instruments introduced into the patient's body through a small, flexible tube, guided by sophisticated optical devices. Because this technique required only a tiny surgical incision, patients experienced substantially less postoperative pain and required far shorter hospitalization and recovery periods. Colonoscopy, the use of a tube inserted into the colon for biopsy and removal of suspicious lesions, also obviated the need for abdominal surgery in many cases. Arthroscopy, using a technique similar to laparoscopy on damaged joints, converted a hospital operation with a long recovery period into a relatively routine outpatient procedure. More recently, techniques using miniaturized instruments introduced through a small incision in the chest have been used to reduce the traumatic consequences of traditional coronary bypass procedures.

The medical benefits of these new noninvasive and minimally invasive techniques were enormous. However, any overall cost saving that might have been expected from fewer hospital admissions, shorter hospital stays, and decreased surgical complications was more than offset by the fact that physicians began performing these procedures on larger and larger numbers of patients who stood to benefit from them but who would not previously have been considered candidates for surgery.

Other therapeutic advances were embraced with equal enthusiasm by the medical profession and its patients. Hips or knees badly damaged by arthritis or fractures could now be replaced, thanks to the introduction of improved materials for artificial joints. Ultrasound machines that use shock waves to break up kidney and gall stones replaced surgery in many instances. Corneal implants to restore vision dimmed by cataracts, coronary bypass grafts to relieve the severe pain of angina, and techniques to reopen narrowed arteries quickly became standard procedures. Transplantation of vital organs and bone marrow opened the way to treatment of previously hopeless diseases. In vitro fertilization as an aid to infertile couples, the gamma knife for noninvasive radiation treatment of brain tumors, and radio-frequency obliteration of arrhythmia-producing nerve pathways in the heart also blazed new paths to improved care.

Infections were treated more effectively by new classes of antibiotics—although drug-resistant organisms emerged as an unexpected challenge to therapy. Drugs for the management of serious diseases such as hypertension, depression, and schizophrenia were developed. Benign enlargement of the prostate, which plagues the majority of men over the age of 65, began to be treated successfully by medication rather than surgery, using one drug that shrinks the prostate and another that relieves the spasm at the neck of the bladder. The incidence of heart attacks and the death rate associated with them were lowered by the use of innovative drugs, as well as by a gradual improvement in American dietary habits and a reduction in smoking.

Although many of the medical advances of the past 25 years involved high technology, some were based on simple, old-fashioned clinical observations that led to departures from previously accepted orthodoxy. One was the discovery that peptic ulcer, once confidently assumed to be caused by psychological stress and the resulting over-production of stomach acids, was in fact caused by the presence of a microorganism that thrives in the stomach. Dr. Barry Marshall, a young physician-in-training in Perth, Australia, noticed odd-looking bacteria in biopsies of inflamed stomach tissues and was struck by the heretical thought that this organism, *Helicobacter pylori*, was not simply a passive resident of the stomach but the culprit responsible for ulcer disease.

Marshall turned to himself as the experimental subject: he ingested a generous quantity of *Helicobacter* and subsequently developed the inflamed stomach and associated symptoms that he expected. This finding, combined with the presence of the organisms in every ulcer patient he examined (except for cases in which aspirin-like drugs were the cause), led him to announce in 1985 that *Helicobacter* was the cause of peptic ulcer. The medical community reacted with skepticism, and only when controlled studies showed that ulcers healed—and usually stayed healed—after antibiotic therapy was his position fully vindicated. The lesson here is that even in an era of high technology, original observations and innovations based on low technology can still make major contributions to the science of medicine.

A NEW ERA OF DRUG THERAPY

The 1980s and 1990s saw a renewed emphasis on drug discovery. In addition to searching for pharmaceutically useful compounds among promising bioactive substances like plant extracts and animal venoms, scientists began using the tools of biochemistry to design drugs from scratch in the laboratory. The key to this approach was the recognition and isolation of cell receptors, proteins that reside either on the outside of the cell or within it and initiate a biological response when specific molecules, known as *ligands*, bind to them. The ability of external surface receptors to be bound by ligands such as circulating hormones provides a way for cells to interact with other cells throughout the body.

Receptor-based drug design focuses on the synthesis of ligands that have the specific ability to bind to a particular type of cell receptor, which is responsible for the drug's therapeutic effect. The better the match between the ligand and the drug's intended receptor sites, the more specific the drug's pharmacological action tends to be and the fewer the side effects resulting from attachment to other receptors. New techniques for synthesizing tens of thousands of experimental drugs, and for isolating and characterizing the structure of specific cell receptors, permit rapid screening of potentially useful agents.

The value of ligands that stimulate particular receptors is well illustrated by sumatriptan, a drug for the treatment of migraine headaches. Sumatriptan stimulates a receptor that leads to the constriction of the dilated blood vessels responsible for the migraine attack and, in the great majority of patients, promptly relieves all symptoms without side effects. Powerful therapeutic effects can also be achieved by agents that block or inhibit normal receptor responses. Ondansetron, a highly effective drug for controlling the nausea and vomiting that plague patients receiving chemotherapy, as well as many postoperative patients, acts by interfering with a specific cell receptor in the central nervous system that causes the muscles in the intestinal wall to go into spasm.

Receptors in the brain are becoming the single largest focus of receptor research. They offer the hope of targeted treatments for obesity, sleep disorders, memory loss, and impotence, as well as a variety of debilitating psychiatric diseases like schizophrenia, obsessive-compulsive disorder, and manic depression. Difficulties arise when receptors specific to a single compound such as serotonin have more diverse effects than scientists anticipated. Prozac (fluoxetine), for example, affects a receptor that keeps serotonin levels in the brain at a therapeutically effective level, but the drug also acts upon a dozen or more other serotonin receptors throughout the body, each of which plays a different role. One influences sexual function; another modifies digestion. Such unwanted receptor responses, constituting adverse side effects, often limit the utility of receptor-targeted drugs. Additional research will be required to design drugs that discriminate between similar receptors in different parts of the body and limit the unwanted side effects of drug therapy.

In 1997, there were reports of a new class of anti-asthma drugs that work by blocking the specific receptors that produce the bronchospasm and resultant breathing difficulty characteristic of an asthmatic attack. And a new drug that targets the receptors responsible for triggering the joint inflammation of rheumatoid arthritis has also raised hope for a better approach to this disabling disease. Some receptor-targeted drugs unfortunately do not keep working indefinitely, since receptors stimulated by a drug over a long period eventually lose their capacity to respond. Attempts to "resensitize" the exhausted receptors and to restore their responsiveness are now at the cutting edge of receptor research.

FIRST FRUITS OF BIOTECHNOLOGY

Another important new class of drugs consists of human proteins manufactured through genetic engineering techniques. Genetic cloning allows for the synthesis of large quantities of proteins, such as hormones, that are identical to the ones produced normally by the body. These proteins can then be administered and used for a variety of therapeutic purposes. A hormone made by the kidney, called erythropoietin, was the first human hormone to be produced in this fashion. It stimulates red blood cell production in the bone marrow and is responsible for maintaining normal red cell levels in the blood. Consequently, patients with extensive kidney damage and a deficiency of erythropoietin typically develop severe anemia. In the past, only repeated transfusions could provide partial control of the problem.

Red blood cell counts in the majority of patients with renal failure can now be maintained at near-normal levels with erythropoietin. Relief from symptoms like weakness and fatigue is usually striking. Erythropoietin has also become a mainstay in controlling the adverse effects of chemotherapy, which typically induces a sharp and sometimes life-threatening reduction in red cell count. Erythropoietin administration makes possible far more aggressive chemotherapeutic regimens for patients who need them. Multiple blood transfusions, with their inherent risks, are much less often needed now as an adjunct to chemotherapy.

White blood cell counts also fall drastically during chemotherapy, increasing the risk of serious infections. This problem has been alleviated by the identification and cloning of the gene that initiates white cell growth through production of so-called "granulocyte colony stimulating factor." This agent has permitted chemotherapy for patients who otherwise might not tolerate it. Similarly, production of the platelet-stimulating factor thrombopoietin is aiding patients with temporary platelet deficiency who are at risk for uncontrolled bleeding.

These naturally occurring hormones, now reproduced in the laboratory, are representative of the first wave of biotechnology-based pharmaceuticals. They are the forerunners of drugs that will not simply reproduce naturally occurring substances in the body, but will instead constitute completely new agents, designed specifically to correct the abnormalities induced by genetically based diseases. Although cloning techniques have already proved their worth at the bedside, they will yield their most important dividends in the decades ahead.

MEDICAL PROGRESS BEHIND THE SCENES

Many of these advances have been featured in newspaper stories and magazine articles because they represent quantitative leaps in medical science. Even the least knowledgeable patient has probably heard about ultrasound and bypass surgery. By contrast, the thousands of small improvements that have collectively transformed medical specialties like anesthesia or neonatal intensive care receive relatively little public attention.

To illustrate this point, it may be helpful to look at the evolution of general anesthesia since the 1950s. The progress of general anesthesia is of more than academic interest because many of us will at some point in our lives experience it, surrendering control of our most basic vital functions—breathing rate, body temperature, hydration, blood pressure, and muscle tone—to the expertise and equipment of the anesthesiologist. Just a few decades ago, the technology to support these functions was relatively primitive, but

striking advances in our understanding of the problems of anesthesia have radically improved the standard of care.

General Anesthesia in 1950 The anesthesiologist in 1950 was a pilot
flying without instruments; success relied on an amalgam of in-
tuition and luck. Lacking reliable tools for monitoring vital signs
during surgery, or for delivering controlled amounts of anesthesia,
the anesthesiologist depended on instinct and unaided observation.
It was, in fact, almost impossible to maintain the patient at a constant level of anesthesia because delivery of the anesthetic gases
was manually controlled. The amount of gas administered in this
way was at best approximate, and could be unexpectedly high or
low depending on the amount of gas remaining in the small storage
tanks. The equally important administration of oxygen to the patient was a similarly rough-and-ready affair. Cardiac arrest or brain
damage were the consequences of failures of this inexact science.

Monitoring of vital signs during surgery consisted mainly of
periodic blood pressure and pulse readings taken with a manual
blood pressure cuff and stethoscope. Tracking the level of blood
oxygenation depended primarily on the anesthesiologist's visual
inspection of the color of the patient's lips, tongue, and fingers.
Body temperature was checked only if the patient's skin was no-
ticeably hot or cold to the touch. As a result, undetected high body
temperature could lead to severe fluid loss and oxygen deficiency;
low body temperature could bring on cardiac arrhythmias.

For doctors and nurses as well as for patients, the operating room
itself could be dangerous. Escape of anesthetic gases into the operating room posed the risks of chemical explosion and of carcin-
ogenic and other toxic effects on operating room personnel. The
explosive potential of anesthetic gases also threatened the patient
in a less direct way by precluding the use of most electrical monitoring equipment, such as the standard electrocardiograph. Rou-

tine reuse of tubing and masks without adequate sterilization increased the risk of nosocomial (hospital-based) infections, especially tuberculosis.

Under the best of circumstances, general anesthesia was a risk, and when human error was added to the equation the patient's chances declined precipitously. Insertion of airway tubes into the esophagus instead of the trachea, for instance, could quickly lead to oxygen deprivation; without automatic monitoring devices such errors could go undetected until the patient's life was endangered. Patient mortality was high during the immediate postoperative period because postoperative recovery units with appropriate physiologic monitoring had not yet been developed. Most surgeries and recoveries, of course, proceeded routinely, but for the patient who started to develop problems, the situation could quickly and inexplicably go from bad to worse.

General Anesthesia in 1970   General anesthesia in 1970 was a far more controlled and safe procedure than it had been only 20 years earlier. Thanks to advancements in chemical and electrical technology, the anesthesiologist now had immediate and continuous access to reliable data on the patient's respiration, blood chemistry, and cardiac activity. Improved equipment permitted more reliable and precisely titrated delivery of anesthetic agents, and the dangers of the immediate postoperative period were more clearly understood and avoided.

The benefits of improved physiologic monitoring began with preoperative screening, in which patients were tested and, if necessary, treated for blood chemical imbalances or other problems that could cause problems during surgery. Such screening was especially valuable for seriously ill patients, who can easily develop imbalances of sodium and potassium in the blood or compromised pulmonary function. Preoperative testing afforded the anesthesiologist a chance to anticipate the problems that the patient could be expected to encounter.

The storage and delivery system for anesthetic gases was vastly improved from the system of portable tanks and tubes that prevailed in 1950. Anesthetic gases were now stored in a central facility of the hospital and were delivered to the operating table through convenient wall plugs. The anesthesiologist had the option of administering gases by means of a mechanical ventilator to patients who could not breathe spontaneously during surgery. Risks to the patient and operating room personnel were further reduced by the introduction of new, nonexplosive anesthetic agents and the use of disposable masks and tubing.

During anesthesia, the patient's vital functions were monitored continuously, with electrocardiography to warn of heartbeat irregularities, blood chemical analysis to track changes in acid-base balance and electrolyte levels, and careful monitoring of blood loss and urine flow to guide fluid replacement measures. By 1970, the patient was no longer taken directly from surgery to a regular hospital room but made an intermediate stop in a recovery area near the operating room. The recovery room was staffed with specially trained nurses who had access to a range of sophisticated equipment and to specialist physicians. It allowed for prompt and effective treatment of unusual but serious post-anesthetic problems such as shock, convulsions, breathing difficulties, and cardiac arrhythmias. Patients who continued to experience serious problems after surgery were sent to the intensive care unit, at that time an innovation in hospital care.

General Anesthesia Today   General anesthesia on the eve of the twenty-first century is characterized by increasingly sophisticated patient monitoring systems and by major advances in the integration and presentation of data to the anesthesiologist. Important progress has been achieved in the monitoring of oxygen levels in the blood, an invaluable indicator of correctly managed patient ventilation during anesthesia. A simple device, called a pulse oximeter, is attached to the patient's finger by a spring clamp and provides continuous readings of both oxygen levels and pulse rate. An alarm sounds if either the pulse rate or oxygen level falls to a dangerously low level. Equally indicative of stable respiration is the level of carbon dioxide exhaled by the patient. CO_2 sensors now show the anesthesiologist the precise concentration of carbon dioxide in each breath. High CO_2 levels warn of inadequate lung ventilation; low CO_2 levels warn of hyperventilation. An absence of CO_2 can indicate that airway tubes have been positioned incorrectly. Heart and circulatory activity now are tracked by devices that provide intermittent or continuous blood pressure readings and electrocardiography. In patients undergoing heart surgery, echocardiography is used to monitor the activity of the heart muscle and valves.

Much of this information is made available to the anesthesiologist in a single data display, so that it can be easily viewed and analyzed. Alarms signal potentially dangerous readings, and the equipment automatically maintains a log of the patient's physiologic status throughout the surgery. In addition, a host of individually minor improvements, such as the ability to control the temperature of transfused blood and the use of hot-air blankets to treat drops in body temperature, together have created a system that is much better equipped to predict and respond to each patient's particular needs.

Postoperative recovery has been made safer by use of the same physiologic monitors. But perhaps the most significant improvement from the patient's point of view has been in the area of postoperative pain management. Until recently, pain medication, such as morphine, was administered intramuscularly at four-hour intervals. After its effect peaked in the first hour or two, the patient might suffer severe pain until the next dose. Now some patients are given the ability to administer their own pain-relieving drugs by means of an infusion pump. Morphine can be administered intravenously at the press of a button, with almost immediate and consistent relief of pain.

In forty years, anesthesia has gone from a largely intuitive art to a well-controlled science based on reliable data and computer-aided analysis. Not surprisingly, these changes have sharply decreased the mortality associated with general anesthesia. The American Society of Anesthesiology reports that the death rate attributable to anesthesia errors has fallen 95 percent just in the last ten years, from 1 to 2 deaths per 10,000 anesthesias to a current rate of 1 death per 200,000 to 300,000 anesthesias. This reduction has been accompanied by fewer malpractice suits and a 50 percent drop in malpractice insurance premiums.[10]

MEDICAL PROGRESS, COSTS, AND THE NATION'S HEALTH

The advances that have occurred within the last twenty-five years are now taken for granted, and their role in driving up costs is generally forgotten. The tendency has been to blame inefficiency and greed in the health care system rather than to face the root issue, namely that advancing technology continually opens up new realms of medical care. During the past two decades new technology has been responsible for approximately half of the 6 percent (inflation-adjusted) annual rise in expenditures on care; the rest is due to rising costs of wages and supplies.[11] Total spending rose to $635 billion in 1995 for doctors, hospitals, and drugs, and the percentage of GDP devoted to health also rose, nearly doubling from 7.4 percent in 1970 to 13.6 percent in 1995.[12] Health care expenditures began to force employers to divert money from wage increases into health insurance premiums and for the first time threatened to bankrupt Medicare and Medicaid programs.

At the same time, the high expenditure on health care in the

United States was—and continues to be—criticized as yielding no obvious benefits as measured by the usual indexes of national health. Lower infant mortality in countries that spend less on health care, for instance, is cited by some as evidence of our inefficiency. Countries such as the United Kingdom, Germany, and the Netherlands, which spend only 7 to 9 percent of their GDP on health care, have infant mortality rates of 6 to 7 per 1,000 live births, compared to 8 per 1,000 live births in the United States.[13] But these arguments are misleading. Many factors other than health care affect infant mortality: poverty and lack of education appear to be the major contributory factors in subgroups of the population with the highest mortality rates.

Average life expectancy at birth in the United States, a second statistic cited to indict the failures of the health care system, is indeed lower in the United States, where it is 76 years, compared to 77 to 78 years in the United Kingdom, Germany, and the Netherlands.[14] But longevity is not the sole measure of quality health care throughout life. Modern, high-tech medicine can extend lives, often in a dramatic fashion, but much of what physicians and hospitals do has primarily increased quality of life, not length of life. Examples abound: angioplasty and coronary bypass procedures that relieve pain without necessarily extending life, hip replacement that increases mobility and reduces pain, lens implants for cataracts (the most common procedure under Medicare) that convert a dim world into one that is bright and clear, and drugs for the treatment of depression and schizophrenia. The ability to provide such care promptly and reliably is almost unique to the United States health care system. Providing care that improves quality of life is a major return on our national investment in health care whether or not it increases average lifespan; it must be taken into account in any debate on the comparative expenditures and effectiveness of health systems.

WHAT'S WRONG WITH SPENDING MORE ON HEALTH CARE?

The extension of health insurance to some 85 percent of the population during the 1960s and 1970s was rightly heralded as an important social advance.[15] Pooling funds to spread the risk and financial burden of expensive care and lengthy hospitalization freed most patients from fear of financial ruin in the event of a serious illness or accident. But such pooling of resources also, understandably, led insured patients to expect the best possible diagnostic and therapeutic care, no matter how expensive the care and how small the expected benefit. This indifference to cost on the part of both physician and patient also extended to hospitals, since their costs for virtually all services were simply passed on to the insurer.

An indemnity-based insurance system (i.e., the old Blue Cross type) obviously encourages high-quality care, but it also invites overuse of services. Although *overuse* is a subjective term, I use it to describe situations in which some portion of the dollars spent are purchasing care for which the costs exceed, and often far exceed, the potential benefits—an expensive antibiotic when a less expensive one could serve almost as well, a longer stay in the hospital that does little to aid recovery, a coronary bypass graft when medications can achieve virtually the same result, and costly cancer chemotherapy when the chances of success are close to zero. Such overuse of services under indemnity insurance plans has contributed significantly to the steep rise in health care costs.

Unlike household fire insurance, the value of which is fixed at the replacement cost of the home or some agreed upon lower value, most indemnity health insurance entitles the insured to benefits with virtually no upper limit. Insurance leads patients and the physicians who act as their agents to use far more health care than they would if they had to pay out of pocket. This is to some extent true of any sort of insurance policy, but the open-ended nature of health insurance coverage leads to expenditures that are especially out of balance with actual benefits to the insured.

The equally sharp rise in expenditures in other sectors of the economy such as consumer electronics raises no similar concerns about excessive spending, at least from the economists' point of view. Consumers are simply making marketplace choices, balancing the perceived benefit of these items against the costs incurred, and trading off the benefits of a cell phone purchase against, perhaps, a new fishing rod. Health care spending, however, represents a much more troublesome phenomenon because insurance blunts the normal cost-restraining mechanisms of the consumer marketplace. As I show in later chapters, one important goal of the switch from indemnity-based to managed care insurance plans was to place some restraints on demand and thereby get the upper hand on expenditure growth. Before the managed care era, however, the cost dilemma was addressed through a flurry of government and insurance industry initiatives aimed at eliminating obviously wasteful practices and at least those aspects of expensive care that were clearly ineffective.

2

Failed Attempts at
Sustained Cost Control

In the early 1980s, the rapid rise in costs of health care suddenly commanded the serious attention of business and government, the two main providers of health insurance. As noted earlier, costs of acute care (hospitals, physicians, and drugs) were rising at an inflation-corrected rate of more than double the 3 percent average annual rise in gross domestic product. Government funds were being soaked up at an alarming rate by Medicare and Medicaid. As a result, new and intensive cost-saving efforts were undertaken, with the main emphasis on reducing hospitalization because hospital charges accounted for the largest portion of acute care expenditures. The most vigorous cost-control efforts in the hospital sector were directed initially to reducing the number of days patients remained in the hospital, eliminating so-called "unnecessary" hospital days. The first to feel the effects of this new strategy were Medicare recipients, but even patients with full insurance soon were subjected to similar efforts.

THE WAR ON HOSPITAL COSTS

The Medicare program set this cost-containment effort into motion in the public sector by introducing a new reimbursement scheme based on so-called diagnosis-related groups (DRGs) in 1983. Before DRGs, hospitals were reimbursed for each component of care—daily room charges, X-ray examinations, laboratory tests, and so forth. Under the DRG system, the government set a single charge as the standard payment for treating any given illness. Charges were based on average costs of caring for that group of patients—regardless of the resources actually expended on a particular patient. This mode of payment provided a major incentive for hospitals to cut short the length of hospital stays. Although it provided no obvious incentive to reduce the number of hospital admissions, the DRG system stimulated a sharp reduction in admissions as well. Serious efforts at implementing DRGs began in 1982. During the years 1984 and 1985, the total number of days patients spent in hospitals fell by 14 percent, and the rate of rise in costs fell sharply from the previous 6 percent annual rate to 2 to 2.5 percent annually.[1] All of the reduction in costs over this brief period can be accounted for by the decrease in hospital days.

This dramatic slowing of the rise in hospital costs was greeted with a heady mixture of optimism and relief by policymakers and insurers, who were convinced they had found the way out of the cost spiral. The smaller increases seemed particularly impressive because they indicated that costs were rising no faster than the general growth in GDP. The secretary of the Department of Health, Education and Welfare, Margaret Heckler, led the parade of celebrants in concluding that "the backbone of the health inflation monster has been broken." To ensure this optimistic outcome, in the decade that followed the government, the insurers, and the hospitals themselves unleashed a host of related cost-containment strategies. The most significant were the practices of "utilization review," closing or merging low-occupancy hospitals, restricting physicians' freedom in prescribing expensive drugs, emphasizing early screening of patients for potential illnesses, and establishing guidelines for standard modes of treatment. The intent of most of these strategies was to ensure that no more resources were expended on the care of a patient than could be medically justified. In other words, the goal was not to deny patients useful care, but simply to eliminate demonstrably inefficient and wasteful practices.

Given the scope and intensity of these efforts, it might have been supposed that the 3 percent inflation rate of the 1984–1986 period could have been sustained or even improved. But something very different happened. Between 1987 and 1992 annual cost increases rose quickly and disconcertingly to an average of nearly 6 percent.[2] It is difficult to generalize about what went wrong with this second wave of cost containment efforts, but it is fair to say that each of the new strategies was flawed in some fundamental ways, and that none of them really came to grips with the fundamental problem: that the universe of medically justifiable interventions was (and is) continuing to expand.

Utilization Review   Utilization review (UR) has been viewed as a key tool for reducing unnecessary hospital days, particularly by eliminating unnecessary admissions. In the late 1980s and early 1990s, it became the cornerstone of efforts to contain expenditures in the private sector. The program rests on the premise that the time a patient spends in the hospital and the resources required to treat that patient should not be determined by the physician alone but should be reviewed by a presumably impartial third party. This third party is typically a representative of the insurer, which has an interest in seeing that costs are kept to a minimum. As cost containment has become the watchword of the health insurance industry, UR has now been instituted in over 90 percent of health plans and has become a prominent feature of the U.S. health care system.[3]

Utilization review can take place at three different points: prior to hospitalization (prospective review), during hospitalization (concurrent review), and after discharge (retrospective review).

Prospective review, or precertification for admission, is the most widely used approach. Employees of the insurer assess the physician's reasons for recommending hospitalization and either approve or deny the request. The reviewers may be registered nurses, licensed practical nurses, pharmacists, or medical technicians. Second opinions from another physician are sometimes sought to determine if an inexpensive surgical procedure can substitute for a more expensive one. Only emergencies are exempt from the precertification process. Prospective review is also now being used to assess the appropriateness of outpatient surgery and diagnostic procedures. One notorious example of precertification, now outlawed by federal regulation, was the one-day limit imposed by some HMOs on hospitalizations for normal childbirth.

Concurrent review is conducted once the patient is in the hospital. The goal is to minimize length of stay and to make plans that will facilitate the patient's timely discharge. *Retrospective review* takes place after the patient is discharged and involves examination of medical records and the associated patient-related charges for the purpose of determining the "medical necessity" of the care that was provided. In some instances, companies will not reimburse for care deemed inappropriate. Other companies simply use the information to "educate" physicians about practices that appear wasteful.

Critics of utilization review object to the process on the grounds that because reviewers, at several removes from the bedside, cannot be aware of all the variables in the case, they are not in a position to make definitive judgments on therapy. Second, the critics argue that the reviewers are not qualified to make professional judgments that override the physician's recommendation. Appeals to a higher administrative level staffed by physicians are usually possible, but these reviewers are also cut off from contact with the patient. The entire process is costly and time-consuming for both payers and providers, and precious time must be spent by physicians in pleading on behalf of their patients. Recent studies on the effectiveness of UR for a sample of health plans suggest that a *one-time* savings of up to 6 percent may be possible when prior authorization and concurrent review programs are instituted together.[4] However, none of the studies of UR have taken into account the providers' costs of administering UR programs, so the net effect on the health system as a whole cannot be calculated.

Controlling the Rise in Drug Costs Controlling the cost of drugs has been one of the focal points in cost-containment efforts. To this end, insurers and hospitals have restricted formularies of approved drugs, with an emphasis on the less expensive generic versions of drugs. Although drug costs are among the most obvious health care costs to the consumer, they constitute only about 10 percent of total acute care spending and thus do not in themselves contain the key to overall cost containment.[5]

Reducing Hospital and Physician Administrative Costs During the last decade, pressures from Medicare and managed care groups, along with competition among insurers, have forced hospitals and physicians to reduce administrative costs through automation, restructuring, and outsourcing of some hospital functions like laundry and food services. Advocates of a Canadian-style, government-run health care system argue that further savings could be achieved if the U.S. adopted a similar approach. However, the studies claiming to support this view have greatly overestimated the potential gain, because they treat a host of essential administrative expenses, like maintaining patient records, as unnecessary. These studies have also deceptively understated costs in Canada by not counting many hidden administrative expenditures.[6]

Closing and Merging Hospitals As a result of cost containment efforts designed to eliminate unnecessary care, the average patient census of U.S. hospitals fell dramatically from 76 percent occupancy in

1981 to 63 percent in 1994.[7] This figure has led to the conclusion that there is a large pool of costly "excess" hospital beds in the United States. In this view the pool of beds in community hospitals represents a waste of scarce resources that could be saved by closing low-occupancy hospitals. The argument is plausible enough on its face, but the fact is that eliminating such empty beds may have almost no effect on overall hospital costs.

Why is this so? Part of the explanation lies in the erroneous assumption that empty beds are always "excess" beds. Deciding what constitutes an excess bed and how many of the empty beds are truly excess is not a simple matter, because empty beds are of two very different types—those that are virtually never used and those that accommodate fluctuation in demand. Because hospitals do not have a constant occupancy rate, they must keep beds available for emergencies and weekly and seasonal variations in demand (occupancy is substantially higher on weekdays than weekends). How large this reserve should be is debatable and very much dependent on what are deemed an acceptable rate of turning away patients during periods of peak demand and acceptable delays before admission. But experience suggests that an 85 percent average occupancy rate is almost certainly the highest that U.S. hospitals could hope to achieve. From this, it follows that there are at most 135,300 "excess" beds in the country as a whole.[8]

Further limiting any savings from eliminating beds is the fact that chronically empty beds impose almost no costs on the system. Such beds make no demand on nursing care, laboratories, food, or supplies—the activities that account for the overwhelming majority of a hospital's expenses. Even closing an entire hospital and transferring its patients elsewhere has little impact on overall costs for a closely related reason: the costs attributable to labor and supplies—some 80 percent of total costs—follow the patient.[9] Thus even the elimination of all excess beds would yield a saving of no more than a few billion dollars in an industry in which total annual costs of community hospitals stood at more than $275 billion in 1994.[10]

Even this relatively modest figure considerably overstates the possible saving. Most of the hospitals that have closed, or are likely to close, are those with the lowest census—typically rural and small urban hospitals. These hospitals are also, by and large, the least sophisticated and the least costly. Transferring their patients to a larger institution that provides more specialized care could well consume whatever modest saving might result from closures. The change of site might be medically beneficial to some patients, but it would not improve the bottom line of the health care system. For other patients, especially those requiring swift emergency treatment for heart attack, stroke, or accidental trauma, closing of local hospitals can be life-threatening.

Reducing the Occurrence of Fraud   The idea of cutting costs by eliminating fraud has enormous appeal—dollars are saved, and wrongdoers who plunder the system are brought to justice. And there is growing evidence that the extent of fraud in the health care system may indeed be large. According to a recent study by federal investigators, some $23 billion in inappropriate charges (accounting for 14 percent of total charges) was billed to Medicare in 1996 alone.[11] What portion of that amount is attributable to differing interpretations of complex regulations or clerical errors, as opposed to deliberate fraud, has not been determined. However, initial reports in 1997 of a federal investigation into Medicare billing practices at the Columbia/HCA Healthcare Corporation, the nation's largest hospital chain, indicated the possibility of a deliberate fraud at a "systemic" level.[12]

Pre-payment and post-payment audits of hospital billings are currently the heart of fraud control strategies, but they have little preventive value; such methods reliably catch honest error but do little to detect criminal fraud.[13] And because the level of fraud is so difficult to track, no one really knows how much effort should be put into fraud control to yield cost-effective results. Although efforts to reduce fraud within the health care system are laudable and necessary, the hope that they might contain the key to long-term control of costs appears to be overly optimistic.

PREVENTIVE MEDICINE AND RATIONAL MODES OF CARE

Two new strategies have been advocated for saving health care dollars while at the same time improving quality of care: encouraging early screening of patients for a variety of potential diseases, and establishing formal guidelines for the standard treatment of common complaints. The question is whether, aside from the probable benefits to patients of these initiatives, they can really save money.

Screening and Preventive Medicine   The proposition that screening of patients for early indicators of disease can reduce health care costs is seductive but overstated. With few exceptions, a screening measure must be applied to large numbers of people in order to save a small number of lives—and often at great expense. Screening for colon cancer is a good example. Colon cancer kills about 50,000 people each year at a cost of about $1 billion in health care.[14] The mortality rate could be reduced sharply, by about 20,000 deaths per year, if a systematic screening program were put in place. An annual test for blood in the stool for the 65 million people over the age of 50 and a colonoscopy for the 10 percent (or 6.5 million) who show a positive result would save many lives. The desirability of pursuing this strategy in the interests of public health are obvious. The fiscal impact is another matter. The total cost of colonoscopy for the 6.5 million candidates would be $4 to $ 6 billion, many times more than the current costs of caring for the 20,000 patients whose cancer could be prevented.[15]

Prevention of disease often falls short of its economic promise because a short-term saving is converted into a much larger long-term cost. Consider heart attacks avoided by a healthier diet, liver failure avoided by lowering consumption of alcohol, and a variety of lethal diseases avoided by smoking cessation. In many cases, a relatively inexpensive death is exchanged for the prospect of even more expensive illnesses in later life, such as Alzheimer's disease, severe arthritis, or pulmonary failure. Treatment for these and other long-term diseases can easily swallow up the savings of earlier efforts at disease prevention. Again, from the patient's standpoint, screening and other tools of preventive medicine are desirable and effective forms of intervention. But, economically speaking, they offer no immediate solution to the problem of rising costs.

Practice Guidelines   Doctors often disagree on the appropriate way to handle a particular clinical situation—for example, whether to order mammograms for women under the age of 50; the desirability of operating on a patient with prostate carcinoma; the extent of surgery that should be done in a woman who has a small area of carcinoma in her breast. Standard "practice guidelines," promulgated by hospitals, government bodies, or professional organizations, have been proposed to avoid inconsistent and possibly wasteful medical care. In establishing them, a panel of experts adopts a consensus recommendation for all practicing physicians governed by the guidelines. These recommendations are often based on systematic studies of clinical outcomes of various forms of treatment, but they ultimately rely on a body of accepted expert opinion. Practice guidelines are being developed for a growing number of illnesses.

The strategy appears eminently reasonable: it promises to improve patient welfare, discourage unnecessary treatment, and save money at the same time. But attractive as it may seem, the obstacles to implementation are substantial and the results unpredictable. Physicians who don't accept the consensus view concerning, for instance, mammography, will find ways to continue in their accustomed mode of practice. In many illnesses, the description of the clinical findings can be slanted sufficiently to justify physicians acting outside the guidelines when they think it appropriate. Changes in modes of treatment over time may also make a guideline obsolete, as has happened in the case of obstruction of the carotid artery in the neck. Not long ago, the established view was that surgery was contraindicated; now it is evident that some types of carotid obstruction are helped substantially by surgery. Guidelines that are overtaken by new knowledge cannot readily be altered, since reestablishing a review committee and analyzing the new data require substantial effort and resources. A recent report from Maine, the first state that has tested practice guidelines for a sustained period (five years), lends credence to doubts about their effectiveness.[16] The study revealed that the protocols have very little impact on physician behavior. Indeed, physicians who have participated in guidelines programs are more pessimistic than their peers about the value of guidelines in improving quality of care and in discouraging the practice of defensive medicine.

The extent to which practice guidelines improve quality of care remains uncertain, as does the amount of money that can be saved. Practice guidelines were intended not only to improve the quality of care, but to eliminate a substantial number of unnecessary and costly procedures. As it has turned out, the guidelines may exert the reverse effect, encouraging modes of treatment that are more expensive than other widely practiced approaches. One of the first sets of practice guidelines released by the federal government, for instance, identified undertreatment of pain as a major problem and called for more aggressive drug treatment, more clinics specializing in pain management, and increased use of alternative therapies like chiropractic.[17] Regardless of identifiable savings, however, practice guidelines *are* serving to educate physicians about evolving medical consensus on treatment options and making them more aware of the cost implications of their decisions.

THE STUBBORN CLIMB IN COSTS: 1987–1992

Despite all the efforts just described, there was, as we have seen, virtually no slowing of the rise in hospital costs between 1987 and 1992. Although total hospital days continued to fall about 2 percent per year the concomitant rise in outpatient visits to hospitals fully offset any inpatient savings.[18] The extraordinary growth in outpatient visits was a function of several developments. One of the most significant was the shift of many routine surgeries to the outpatient setting. This shift saved little money because the most significant costs of treatment—physicians' fees, nurses and other support staff, and operating room supplies—are the same whether or not the patient is admitted overnight. Only the cost of the hospital's "hotel" functions is saved.

Ambulatory visits also grew as a result of earlier discharges from the hospital for those patients who did manage to get admitted. Much of the saving from the shrinking average length of stay was thus offset by the costs of the additional follow-up visits to the hospital required for the discharged patients. Generally unaccounted for are the additional costs of follow-up care outside the hospital in doctors' offices and the costs of in-home care necessitated by early discharges from the hospital.

GLIMMER OF HOPE OR CALM BEFORE THE STORM: 1993–1996

Beginning in 1993, there once again appeared to be a ray of hope in the battle to contain health care costs. After an average increase in hospital costs of nearly 6 percent per year during the previous five years, the rate of increase fell to 4 percent in 1993 and dropped to about 1 percent in 1994 and 1995. This change reflected a reduction in inpatient days of 2.3 percent in 1993, 4.0 percent in 1994, and 3.5 percent in 1995.[19] The rate of increase in outpatient visits remained basically unchanged from the previous five-year period. Lending further support to the hope that a corner had been turned was a leveling off of health insurance premiums. Where did this relief come from, and can the forces responsible for it be expected to have a long-term effect on the rise in costs?

The moderation in insurance premiums was at least partially attributable to the willingness of insurers to sacrifice profits temporarily in an attempt to increase market share. One major organization reported a reduction in profits from 9 percent in 1995 to 4.5 percent in 1996. This type of sacrifice is obviously not intended as a long-term strategy. Some of the other improvements in the cost picture may have come from new efficiency savings, although the source of such savings is as yet unexplained. As discussed earlier, an efficiency saving lowers the cost base once, but does little or nothing to suppress the rise in costs in the long term.

Another significant factor in the moderation of cost increases—and especially of insurance premiums—was the increase in copayments and deductibles that insurers have instituted to discourage use of services and that have shifted an increased portion of financial responsibility to the patient. Whenever the price of goods or services is increased, consumption of at least some services decreases, especially among those least able to pay. It seems unlikely, however, that cost-sharing has been the predominant factor in reducing costs. The reason is that most expenditures on health care are generated by a very small number of extremely sick patients—only 5 percent of the population accounts for half of annual expenditures on health care—and all of these patients quickly pass their copayment limits, thereafter being unaffected by cost-sharing requirements.[20]

Perhaps most significant, costs were held down by eliminating some benefits from insurance packages altogether and by applying stricter standards of acceptance to potential enrollees faced with high-risk illnesses. Denying enrollees some forms of expensive care (certain transplants, for example) by designating the therapies as experimental has also been a cost saver. In such strategies, however, the line between eliminating wasteful spending and denying useful care is almost certainly being crossed.

Indeed, denial of potentially useful care under the rubric of cost effectiveness probably in itself accounts for a large fraction of the slowing of overall hospital expenditures seen between 1993 and 1995. The dramatic reduction in hospital days, particularly because it was not accompanied by a rise above the historic rate of increase in outpatient visits, provides the most compelling evidence that an overall reduction in services accounted for most of the savings. These data suggest that patients are simply getting less care. Lending further credence to this conclusion are the well-publicized reports of enforced early discharges from the hospital after childbirth (and even after such drastic procedures as mastectomy), and "gag rules" restricting managed care physicians from discussing expensive therapies with patients.

Savings due to recent sacrifices in insurer profit margin are clearly not sustainable, and to the extent that they force smaller companies to merge or be forced out of the market, they could in the long run increase costs by reducing competition. Indeed, health care analysts in late 1997 predicted that premiums would rise sharply in 1998. Mark Psleger, director of marketing for the Blue Cross Blue Shield Association, estimated an overall increase of 5 to 10 percent. Small companies, especially those with older employees or employees prone to illness, could be due for increases of as much as 30 percent, according to industry analysts.[21] The first firm number for 1998 is an 8.5 percent increase in health care premiums for federal workers. This increase bodes ill for private sector workers because the Office of Personnel Management is predicting that the federal increase will be significantly lower than the private sector increase, as has historically been the case.[22]

Large savings due to further reductions in total days of hospitalization appear unlikely, since hospitals are already admitting and keeping only the sickest patients, and transferring any more patients to the outpatient sector will have increasingly obvious effects on quality of care. A growing and organized resistance among patients to early hospital discharges demonstrates that further reductions in length of hospital stays will not be tolerated by the public.

Some additional efficiency gains may emerge from computerization of patient records and online submission of insurance claims. Further savings are theoretically possible by eliminating *all* remaining inefficiencies in the health care system, but in the real world perfect efficiency is never attained. And even if half of the potential efficiency gains that have been discussed here were actually achieved (an unlikely possibility), the effect on rising costs would be small, less than 1 percent per year if spread over the next few years.[23] Once such savings are exhausted and can no longer offset the underlying rise in costs, the true rate of rise will once again emerge as it did after the 1984–85 period of respite.

Put differently, virtually every cost-saving measure examined in this chapter does only one thing: it reduces the *level* of spending but does not control the long-term upward *trend* in spending due chiefly to advancing medical technology. For this reason, such savings can produce only a temporary slowing in cost increases. Thus we may have reached the end of the line for efforts at cost containment that target only unnecessary care and administrative waste. Renewed efforts at cost control will step further across the line into denying access to some forms of potentially useful care to some or all patients. And the mechanisms for the next stage of cost control are already emerging in the reorganization of the health care power structure that is currently reshaping the face of American medicine.

THE FORGOTTEN SIDE OF
THE HEALTH CARE SECTOR: NON-ACUTE CARE

Almost all attempts to address rising health care costs have focused on the provision of acute medical care in hospital settings—despite the fact that some 43 percent of total heath care costs in the U.S. are attributable to non-acute care (NAC).[24] Only nursing home care, the single largest component of non-acute care, and home health care, the fastest growing component of NAC, have attracted any sustained interest on the part of policymakers, and because cutbacks on government reimbursements for these services are political dynamite, serious cost containment efforts have been lacking. Additional components of NAC include such diverse sectors as dentistry, over-the-counter drugs and sundries, optometry and other professional services, public health programs, and various administrative costs. Taken together, the average rate of rise for the entire non-acute sector has been about 6 percent in real terms over the last 10 or 15 years, a rate similar to that of the acute sector. It is this combination of rises in both acute and non-acute care that has led to the rise in health care's share of gross domestic product to a level of 14 percent in 1994.

The steep rate of rise in expenditures on non-acute health services may at first seem surprising, since the non-acute sector might be supposed less vulnerable than the hospital-based sector to the inflationary effects of technology. However, many other factors are having inflationary effects on non-acute care, and these factors may be as stubbornly resistant to containment as the advancing state of medical technology is. Ironically, one of the most important factors is an indirect fallout from the dramatic advances in acute care medicine. Because new medical treatments are improving control of many diseases but not providing a complete cure, the growing number of patients who live with chronic diseases is driving a corresponding growth in demand for non-acute care.

Based on research that I conducted along with Daniel Mendelson and Kellie Mitra of the Lewin Group, a health care consulting firm, there appears to be no near-term prospect for a downturn in the rate of growth in NAC expenditures. To illustrate some of the factors that went into our analysis, the examples of nursing home care, home health care, dental care, and over-the-counter drugs are discussed below.

Nursing Home Care (18 Percent of NAC Spending)   Nursing homes are being faced with sicker and sicker patients, as measured by the level of patients' functional impairment, limitations in their activities of daily living, and the number of services that need to be provided for them. This trend will continue in the coming years due to (1) patients being discharged earlier from hospitals, (2) the overall aging of the general population, and (3) the availability and viability of home care for the healthier patients. Also, payment policies of both private and public sector providers will increasingly encourage the use of nursing facilities in place of hospitals for sub-acute care, and the growing popularity of long-term care insurance will make extended nursing home care an option for more and more patients. Given these policies, as well as intense political pressures to sustain government funding under Medicaid, it is hard to envision expenditure increases slowing in the years ahead.

Home Health Care (6 Percent of NAC Spending)   Because it is viewed as a cost-effective alternative to expensive acute and long-term nursing home care, spending on home health care has grown faster than spending in any other sector, increasing an average of 16 percent annually between 1980 and 1993. Growth has been particularly high between 1989 and 1993—some 23 percent annually—fueled by a combination of Medicare and private spending. Technological advances have stimulated the demand by allowing home care agencies to deliver high-technology care, such as parenteral/enteral nutritional therapy, respiratory therapy, chemotherapy, intravenous administration, and hemodialysis. The growth in insurance coverage for home care and payment policies that shift care away from hospitals and nursing homes have also fueled spending growth.

Although the recent double-digit increases in home health care expenditures may represent a one-time spurt, the slowing of that growth in the foreseeable future is uncertain. The Health Care Financing Administration has estimated that home health spending will increase by only 7 percent annually between 1996 and 2002, but it is equally likely that the drive to discover cost-effective substitutes for inpatient care will continue to spur increases at a substantially higher rate unless regulations limiting reimbursement for services provided under Medicare and Medicaid are tightened.

Dentistry (10 Percent of NAC Spending) Although water fluoridation and improved dental care have resulted in a sharp drop in the incidence of dental caries, a variety of new dental services are taking up the slack in dentists' practices. Expanding areas of treatment include cosmetic dentistry, tooth implants, and the application of sealants and veneers. As growing numbers of older Americans retain their teeth longer, they will require additional dental care services. A continued expansion of dental insurance coverage will create an increased demand for services, which will translate into higher total costs.

Over-the-Counter Preparations (7 Percent of NAC Spending) More and more drugs are making the move from prescription to nonprescription status, resulting in steadily growing sales. Examples of prescription drugs that have recently become available over-the-counter include ibuprofen, hydrocortisone, cimetidine (Tagamet), and several antifungal agents. The number of drugs available over the counter is expected to grow in response to the increased interest of consumers in self-medication. Like the substitution of non-acute care for acute care, the switch of a drug from prescription to OTC status may seem like a cost-saver but could actually add to total costs. Sales of a drug rise when patients can buy it without a prescription. The combination of an increased volume of sales and sometimes a higher price for the OTC product than for a generic version bought by prescription can cause total expenditures to rise.

The Outlook   Non-acute care is a growth industry, and costs will continue to drive up total health care costs. It will continue to generate almost half of the nation's overall health care bill. Although the range of predicted rise, from 5 to 8 percent, is relatively wide, the basic conclusion seems clear that non-acute health care costs will continue to grow faster than inflation and that non-acute care will be just as resistant to effective cost control as the acute care sector.

3

Reorganization of the
Health Care Delivery System

We are witnessing a major restructuring of the U.S. health care system—how it is paid for, who delivers it, who controls it—and the pace of change will accelerate in the near future. These changes are reshaping many of the features that Americans have come to take for granted in their health care system. Managed care, the new mantra of health care delivery, is designed to control the costs of care by eliminating unnecessary services. The most visible and familiar form of managed care is the health maintenance organization (HMO), which combines delivery and financing of health services in a single system. HMOs typically provide an extensive package of services for a fixed annual fee. Other common forms of managed care include preferred provider organizations (PPOs), groups of providers such as hospitals and physicians that agree to accept discounted payments from insurers and employers, and independent practice associations (IPAs), usually groups of physicians who band together to contract with insurers or HMOs. Such organizations are replacing traditional fee-for-service arrangements between health-care providers and insurers. Their total membership is growing rapidly and has already reached close to 75 percent of the insured population.[1]

The distinction between managed care plans and traditional indemnity insurance plans is becoming blurred as managed care plans allow patients greater flexibility in choice of physicians and hospitals and as indemnity plans increasingly constrain patient and physician freedom of action through utilization review and other cost-containment measures. One hybrid form, the point-of-service (POS) plan, combines features of both. Under such plans, patients can go outside a contracted provider list to any physician or hospital, so long as they are willing to pay some predetermined portion of the charges, typically 20 percent.

The corporatization of health care also continues to gain momentum as more health care providers join the for-profit sector, and mergers between providers create ever-larger health care corporations. The expressed purpose of these changes is to tap into the competitive efficiencies and capital resources of the for-profit sector. But the more immediate motivation for managed care organizations and hospitals is to retain market share in the face of fierce competition and intense pressure from employers and other payers to hold down premiums. How successful their conversion from charitable to money-making enterprises will be and what the effects will be on quality of care are uncertain. What does seem certain is that an increasing portion of dollars flowing through the system will be earmarked for the executive salaries and stockholder dividends that are part and parcel of for-profit corporations.

THE GROWING DOMINANCE OF MANAGED CARE

In the past health care providers were reimbursed by insurers on a fee-for-service basis. In the new world of managed care, payment is typically based on terms imposed by managed care contracts. In the fee-for-service model, the physician's and hospital's financial incentives were in line with the professional obligation to provide the best possible care for a patient; managed care, by contrast, provides a direct financial incentive for physicians and hospitals to do less for patients, since they typically share some of the risk with the insurer for costs that exceed the target amount. This new model has fundamentally changed the health care system by shifting the balance of power and authority away from physicians and hospitals in favor of insurers. In addition, as managed care organizations assume the double role of insurer and provider, they are in a position to control costs by restricting care.

Under competitive pressures, managed care organizations will begin to distinguish themselves by price and by the range of services they provide. The lowest-priced plans will restrict access to certain expensive procedures, such as heart and liver transplants, and the highest-priced will provide the widest possible range of services, including so-called point-of-service options. Increasing numbers of businesses are now offering their employees a choice of several managed care plans, and these plans must compete for membership based on the combination of price and services they provide.

The verdict is still out on the overall effect of managed care on the nation's health, and I examine some of managed care's more worrisome features in chapter 6. For the moment, according to Dr. Allan Hillman, Professor of Health Policy at the University of Pennsylvania, "Most patients without complex medical problems appear to be well satisfied by managed care services, but with the very sick and those with rare and expensive illnesses, the situation is generally different. . . . Eighty-five percent of medical care is routine and the plans take care of that readily. The gaps in HMOs exist in the less routine situations. And of course the good organizations seek to plug them, but it can take years."[2]

LINKUP OF PROVIDERS

The structure of provider organizations is also changing dramatically with the formation of more highly integrated groups. Across all major sectors of the health care system (including physicians, hospitals, pharmaceutical companies, nursing homes, and home health services), providers are joining forces to form new and larger organizations that they hope will be capable of delivering a wide range of services at lower costs. Whether this promise will be fulfilled is not yet clear. Monopolistic practices may actually increase costs and simply add to the profits of providers.

The linkup of similar providers (horizontal integration) has been expanding rapidly and will continue through the next decade. Hospitals are merging, physicians are combining to form very large group practices, and home health care providers are joining forces. Here again, it is not yet clear whether larger organizations are necessarily more efficient, and whether the efficiency gains that are achieved will be translated into lower costs to the patient, rather than be channeled into higher corporate profits.

The linkup of different types of providers (vertical integration) is also moving forward quickly. This trend is based in the merger of different types of providers into organizations capable of providing a range of different services—from acute care to skilled nursing home care, as well as pharmacy and laboratory services. Integrated providers gain efficiency by reduced administrative and billing costs. Integration also facilitates information exchange throughout the system so that, for instance, requests for blood tests can be transferred to the laboratory electronically rather than on paper, and the results can be transmitted with similar efficiency. Furthermore, data on laboratory use by individual physicians is easily obtainable and allows the managed care organization to monitor utilization patterns. As links are broadened by the integration of medical organizations, laboratories, and drug companies, providers believe they can more closely control unnecessary lab tests, excessive X-rays and other diagnostic imaging, and unwarranted prescriptions. The first wave of integration has already occurred, and competition will force other organizations to follow suit. Independent hospitals and independent laboratories will, in many instances, be forced out of business.

Integration will fundamentally reshape the health care system; these changes may be for the better, but they will not develop without growing pains. Legal and ethical issues are creating significant problems for integrated health care organizations. For example, Merck & Company's acquisition of the health care provider Medco has been investigated by the government to see if Merck is gaining unfair advantage in the pharmaceutical market. In at least one instance, it has been shown that Medco eliminated a number of popular products made by other companies from the list of preferred drugs, including cholesterol-lowering drugs that compete with Merck's products. More recently, Zeneca, the world's second largest manufacturer of cancer drugs, bought out a chain of 11 cancer centers in prestigious U.S. hospitals, including Cedars Sinai in Los Angeles and St. Vincent's Medical Center in Manhattan. Commenting on the obvious potential for conflict of interest in such arrangements, medical ethicist Arthur Caplan commented, "Having your doctor, your clinic, your pharmacy, and your testing lab all owned by the same person is not the optimal structure for health care."[3]

MERGERS OF UNIVERSITY HOSPITALS

A similar attempt to enhance market position through integration of organizations is taking place at the very top of the health-care system hierarchy—the prestigious university-affiliated hospitals. In the last several years, there has been a spate of mergers, sometimes in the face of impending fiscal crisis. Two recent mergers include those of distinguished institutions: the Massachusetts General Hospital and the Brigham and Women's Hospital in Boston, and the New York University Hospital and Presbyterian Hospital in New York. In public statements, the point is made that such mergers will help contain costs. And if a merger involves closing one hospital and moving the patients to the other, building and administrative costs (about 20 percent of total hospital expenditures) may well be lowered. But if both buildings are kept open, as in the mergers just described, these savings will be substantially reduced. On the other hand, mergers that combine the purchasing power of two large university hospitals do provide the resulting institution with far greater power to extract the lowest possible price from suppliers. Some cuts in costs can also be gained in support areas such as marketing, public relations, and computer services, but the overall effect on operational costs of these savings is generally conceded to be modest.

The main advantage of these mergers appears to lie in maintaining or increasing market share. Managed care companies negotiating hospital contracts cannot divide and conquer as easily when confronted with two top-tier university hospitals and their affiliates acting as a unified health care system. The combined hospitals command the allegiance of enough referring physicians to ensure an increasing flow of patients—thereby enhancing market share at the expense of other hospitals in the area. The new 800-pound gorilla can thus drive hard bargains with third-party payers when they negotiate contracts. As cost pressures on merged hospitals continue, the next step is likely to be elimination of expensive, unprofitable services such as burn units. What will happen to patients cared for in such units is a legitimate source of concern. In these cases, the saving to the hospital may simply shift the financial burden to the public sector, resulting in no net saving in system-wide costs.

DISEASE MANAGEMENT

The new "disease management" approach to coordinating health services for particular diseases has an obvious appeal: the promise of lower costs and higher quality care in the integrated treatment of individual serious illnesses. In the traditional care of complex diseases like diabetes, the patient is seen in many different settings (the hospital, various physicians' offices, the nutrition clinic, the podiatry center, etc.), with all care providers playing separate, uncoordinated roles. Disease management shifts the emphasis by consolidating all aspects of care for a given disease through centralized facilities and a specialized team that provides a comprehensive, integrated form of care—from prevention to critical care, and from hospital to home. Health care providers see an opportunity not only to improve care but also, more important from their point of view, to improve efficiency and cut costs.

The illnesses that are most likely to be "carved out" (i.e., separately contracted) in employer-funded health plans are chronic diseases that are expensive to treat: diabetes, asthma, cancer, Alzheimer's disease, stroke, severe spinal and head injuries, and major mental health problems. The more widespread a particular disease, the more likely it is to be a candidate for the disease management approach. A recent survey, for example, found that, in 1995, 42 percent of employer-funded health plans carved out pharmacy benefits, and 20 percent carved out mental health benefits.[4]

Pharmaceutical companies have been the leaders in developing such programs, and many of the conventional managed care providers have sought them out to put a program in place. Nearly all of the pharmaceutical firms engaged in disease management appear to be using the program for a marketing advantage in stimulating drug sales. They therefore design treatment programs that can be expected to make substantial use of their own proprietary products. Some preliminary data suggest that disease management programs can be useful in reducing costs, but their effects on quality of care remain to be definitively demonstrated.

EFFECTS OF HEALTH CARE REORGANIZATION ON ACCESS TO CARE

Given the prevailing political philosophy that favors market forces over egalitarianism, and the increasing role of for-profit organizations in the health care arena, the quality of health care in America will become more and more stratified according to price. At the very least, we can anticipate the evolution of four tiers of medical care entitlement in place of the two (the insured and the uninsured) with which we are familiar.

The first tier will consist of consumers with sufficient income to buy coverage far more comprehensive than the standard package offered by most managed care companies. Their premiums will cover an expensive and sophisticated package of "luxury" services such as MRI scans as part of the annual physical exam, and liberal use of other high-tech procedures. Some of the affluent may decide, in addition, to purchase an option that allows unrestricted choice of doctors and hospitals, perhaps subject to some kind of copayment. The second tier will consist of average citizens who choose a standard managed care package. Their insurance will exclude (in the fine print) some expensive, valuable services. The third tier will consist of the poor who have Medicaid coverage that entitles them to some minimum standard of care, subject to continuing pressure from politicians to keep services at only a barebones level. The fourth tier will consist of the uninsured who do not qualify for Medicaid and who will depend on municipal hospitals, charity facilities, or free clinics for care.

This four-tier structure virtually guarantees that there will be wide disparities in the type and quality of care available to individuals of different financial means. There certainly does not appear to be any practical way to prevent the wealthy from purchasing the kinds of high-cost, marginal-benefit services that will be unavailable, even under the most generous health plans, to the great majority of Americans. At the other end of the spectrum, it seems shameful to many, including myself, that ours is the only advanced nation that does not guarantee health coverage to all its people, including those unable to pay. Care for this segment of the population comes primarily from charitable facilities like neighborhood free clinics. Because the level of services in these settings is generally far below that in the private sector, a deplorable inequity in health care has evolved. It remains to be seen what degree of disparity in levels of medical care will be tolerated before the public demands government intervention to guarantee basic health care rights.

MANAGED CARE AND PHYSICIANS

Patients are by no means the only ones who are being affected by the sweeping reorganization of the U.S. health care delivery system. Health care professionals, and physicians in particular, are finding themselves in a world with completely new rules, increased constraints, and curtailed prerogatives. Constraints on payment under Medicare and Medicaid and limitations on salaries imposed by managed care providers mean that the days of dependable annual increases in physicians' income are over. Many physicians will face flat incomes over the years to come, and more than a few have already seen substantial reductions in earnings.

One might anticipate that this new financial reality, compounded by managed care's control over doctors' professional lives, would discourage applications to medical school. On the contrary, in the mid-1990s applicants have risen to a record high of 45,000.[5] The probable reasons are these: first, alternative professional careers, such as education, law, and business administration, have been similarly affected by decreased earnings expectations and job security; second, the new generation of young physicians is less troubled by the prospect of lower income than their elders because their income losses are partially offset by a more regular work schedule with fewer hours and a greater chance for a fulfilling family life; and third, even as the medical profession loses some of its entrepreneurial allure, it continues to attract altruistic individuals in search of a career that combines intellectual stimulation with the emotional and spiritual rewards of service to others. However, the grim job outlook for medical specialists has recently led to a decline in those pursuing specialist training; more than 50 percent of medical school graduates are applying for primary care training, as compared to only 38 percent a few years ago.[6]

As the demand for physicians falls in the cost-conscious world of managed care, graduates of foreign medical schools (officially known as "international medical graduates" or "IMGs") will add to the physician surplus and will be viewed by U.S.-trained physicians as unwelcome competitors.. To help control this problem, a group of major national medical organizations, including the Association of American Medical Colleges (AAMC) and the Association of Academic Health Centers, issued a "consensus statement on the physician work force." It recommends that the number of positions for residency training be reduced to a level only slightly higher than the number required to accommodate American graduates.[7] (At present, there are about 25,000 first-year residency slots available each year, with about 25 percent of them filled by IMGs. Only about 20 percent of these IMG residents are U.S. citizens).[8]

In a farther-reaching initiative, a coalition of medical educators and doctors have called for a direct restriction on the number of graduates of foreign medical schools who are allowed to train and practice in the United States.[9] Attracted by the high standards and high income of U.S. medicine, physicians who are graduates of non-U.S. medical schools now make up almost 165,000 or 24 percent of practicing physicians in the United States.[10] Whether IMGs are less competent than U.S. graduates is difficult to ascertain, but studies have shown that the frequency of malpractice claims against IMGs is no higher than that of their U.S.-trained colleagues.[11] The prospect that a cutback in IMGs will exacerbate the shortage of doctors in inner-city and rural areas has been a source of concern, but the President of the AAMC, Jordan J. Cohen, has stated that "simply continuing to flood the country with excess physicians, the vast majority of whom wind up in suburbia, will not do."[12]

The perceived problem of a physician surplus is already leading to actions designed to reduce the supply of American graduates as well as of IMGs. It has been recommended that the number of medical students be reduced by 20 percent. Further, the federal government is implementing a program in which teaching hospitals will continue to get subsidies for residency programs even if they substantially reduce the number of residencies available. In other words, they will be paid for not training residents.[13]

WHAT KIND OF SYSTEM IS EMERGING?

These trends all indicate fundamental changes in the system for delivery of health care in the United States. Some key developments to watch for in the coming years are these:

- The health care system will be dominated by fewer and larger providers.
- Corporate interests will have a more important role in the delivery process.
- There will be growing financial incentives to eliminate remaining unnecessary care.
- The federal government will exert increasing pressure on providers to hold down Medicare and Medicaid costs.
- There will be at least four levels of care, as determined by a patient's financial resources.
- Physicians will find themselves in conflicting roles as advocates of patients and employees of cost-conscious provider organizations.

This increasingly competitive and profit-driven environment will have an enormous effect on the way that limited health care resources are allocated—who is cared for, and what kind of care they receive. Increased competition among providers can encourage the elimination of inefficiencies, but competition cannot control the pressure on costs imposed by an ever-expanding arsenal of new technology. Competition can force a hospital to offer a lower-than-average price to a valued buyer such as a large HMO, but some other payer has to make up the shortfall in order for the hospital to avoid fiscal disaster. Once increased competition squeezes out any remaining inefficiencies in the system, it can produce further savings only when competing providers begin to impose serious restrictions on the availability and quality of care offered.

Part Two

Utopian Promise and
Real-World Problems
at the Dawn of the
Twenty-First Century

Part 2 of this book looks forward to the opening years of the next millennium. It focuses on a few of the many areas in which medical progress will be staking out new frontiers and, at the same time, creating new fiscal headaches. Bioengineering advances and a wave of novel drugs designed to target cellular receptors will have the most immediate impact, but the developing power of molecular biology will also play an important role. In particular, the identification and localization of genes associated with particular diseases will give rise to new and sophisticated diagnostic techniques.

This portion of the book also considers various forms of rationing as a means of dealing with cost pressures. Rationing health care to control costs is already a feature, in practice if not in theory, of government-run systems in many European countries. In the United States, the growing ability of managed care organizations and other health insurance providers to control the terms of health care delivery will have a similar effect in the coming decades. As a result, a widening gap between what is medically possible and what is medically customary will create widespread conflicts between patients and health care providers, which will ultimately require resolution in legislatures and the courts. The first skirmishes in this war are already under way.

The pages ahead create a framework for thinking about how our lives might be affected by the coming advances in medical technology and about how an optimal tradeoff between medical progress and cost containment might be achieved. The nation as a whole will be confronted with a difficult choice: to continue fostering the use of technologically advanced techniques and accept a steady, painful rise in health care expenditures, or to limit the availability of these techniques to contain costs. Another policy option would be to deliberately hobble the medical research and development apparatus by cutting back on federal research support. None of these choices appears at the moment to be politically acceptable and, as a result, the nation's leaders continue to indulge in the fading hope of finding painless solutions to the cost problem.

4

Medical Progress in

the Near Term:

2000 to 2020

The decade or two ahead of us will be a transitional period in which many of the engineering techniques of the past two decades are perfected and new ones, targeted at cellular and subcellular processes, make their debut. In particular, molecular medicine will begin to exploit the critical role genes play in human health and disease. The era of bioengineering will reach its zenith in areas like improved (and in many instances miniaturized) instrumentation, novel uses of synthetic biological materials, laboratory production of human tissue using cell culturing techniques, and progress toward artificially intelligent computers that assist in clinical decisionmaking. Molecular medicine in these decades will only begin to fulfill its revolutionary potential, and will do so predominantly in the areas of diagnosis and genetic screening. It will almost certainly take longer for a full range of, useful therapeutic interventions to develop; I consider these in the final chapters of the book. In the near term, the fruits of both bioengineering and molecular medicine will offer interim solutions to clinical problems: sophisticated and effective tools for mitigating the effects of disease and repairing its destructive consequences, but not yet the means of derailing disease at its genetic origins. The paragraphs that follow sketch only a handful of the hundreds of ways in which these advances will enhance patient care in the opening years of the next millennium.

Fast CT and MRI   Accurate images of the beating heart are still beyond the reach of radiologic techniques, but increases in the sophistication of CT and MRI scanners will make them a reality. At present, CT and MRI scanners can obtain precise images only of a motionless object, but future machines operating at high speed will allow the motion of the heart and other physiological processes to be captured in a smooth series of sharp images. Refinements in these methods will make it possible, for instance, to detect coronary artery disease in its early stages, when preventive measures can be taken. Fast magnetic resonance imaging will also be used to detect lung cancers too small to be detected by current techniques. Early detection significantly improves the chances of a cure. Given the frequency of lung cancer and the tragically low cure rate with chemotherapy and radiation, the prospect of earlier diagnosis and intervention is heartening.

Positron Emission Tomography (PET)   Positron emission tomography offers a new radiologic technique for studying the metabolism and biochemistry of cells—often a substantial improvement over the anatomical images obtainable from MRI. After injection of a radioactive compound, PET tracks the metabolic behavior of the injected material. This technique is particularly useful in the study of drug effects on cell function. PET may also afford an early and accurate diagnosis of many diseases, such as cancer and mental illnesses, including Alzheimer's disease, and should allow physicians to precisely assess responses to treatment. At present PET is still largely confined to the research laboratory because of the enormous capital investment that is required and the daunting operational costs. But its eventual role in the clinical arena is virtually assured.

Combining MRI and PET to Study Cell Function　The wedding of MRI with PET scanning has emerged as one of the most promising areas of bioengineering research. MRI can produce elegantly defined renditions of an organ's anatomy, and PET can be used to assess the metabolic function of cells. Uniting the anatomical and biochemical information provided by the two technologies has obvious potential, but it has so far proved impractical because the powerful magnetic fields of the MRI equipment render useless the much more sensitive electronic receivers of the PET scanner. If these problems can be solved, the time may soon be at hand when the physical and metabolic reaction of specific brain regions to drugs or to particular cognitive processes can be assessed simultaneously—and substantially enhance our understanding of brain function.[1]

Coherence Interferometry　Coherence interferometry provides detailed images of the top few millimeters of a given organ by capturing the faint light that is reflected off the tissue. Preliminary studies suggest that the degree of detail can come close to that which is now obtained with biopsy tissue. "Optical biopsies" will open a wide range of noninvasive diagnostic possibilities for organs whose surfaces are readily accessible—eye, colon, and coronary arteries, among others. They will be particularly useful in the diagnosis and management of glaucoma and retinal disease.

Virtual Reality　Work now in progress suggests that it will soon be standard practice to employ computer-generated "virtual reality" as a means of exploring internal body organs.[2] The technique uses digital imaging to recreate the three-dimensional appearance of body structures by synthesizing data from a variety of imaging methods like MRI, CT, and ultrasound. The result is a virtual "peep-hole" into the inner recesses of the body, a tool that is already being used to help surgeons navigate through the complex structures of the brain to eradicate tumors without damaging any of the adjacent tissue. It is also being tested as an alternative to colonoscopy procedures, which require sedation and insertion of a flexible viewing tube into the rectum and colon. By exploring a three-dimensional re-creation of the patient's bowel based on a series of CT images, the physician may be able to sight suspicious growths just as well as by visual colonoscopy.[3] Virtual reality techniques may also provide a supplement to the surgically inserted, miniature cameras that are used to guide laparoscopic and arthroscopic surgery. By supplementing the imaging data with data that reflect the physical and tactile properties of anatomical structures, scientists can re-create the surgeon's experience of an actual procedure. Viewing a three-dimensional re-creation of the surgical site, the cybersurgeon manipulates a scalpel-like equivalent of a joystick and receives feedback on his actions through a virtual-reality headpiece and a glove that simulates tactile responses.

Chemistry Laboratory on a Chip   Conventional laboratories may soon face competition from laboratories built on a single computer chip. Many of the large machines now used to carry out laboratory assays will be replaced by miniaturized circuitry that allows microscopic versions of chemical tests to be performed with almost no human intervention. The devices will accept complex biological samples and automatically perform analyses in seconds and with only tiny volumes of chemical reagents. They promise to improve sensitivity, reliability, and speed of analyses, and to permit use at the patient's bedside, in the home, in doctors' offices, and in remote locations.

CLINICAL COMPUTING AND TELEMEDICINE

The power of the computer and the ubiquity of global Internet connections are turning the global village into a global clinic. Medical records, X-rays, and other diagnostic images will increasingly be created in or translated into digitized form, making them immediately available not only at their place of origin, but wherever else they are needed. The growing practice of telemedicine puts this technology to work by allowing specialist physicians to consult on the treatment of patients hundreds of miles away. Military planners are already working on taking this a step further. They envision that a combination of telecommunications, virtual reality techniques, and robotics will one day allow soldiers in a battle zone to be operated on by a surgeon back home.[4]

One negative side of computerized patient information is, of course, the potential for invasion of patient privacy. The proliferation of data banks in hospitals, hospital networks, managed care organizations, drug companies, and insurance firms has already led to medical records being bought and sold without control by effective government regulations. Some credit card companies and other types of information gatherers are extending their reach into the medical records business, selling the information to drug companies and HMOs.

Computers that make use of "artificial intelligence" techniques to emulate the process of human reasoning have long been considered potentially important tools for analyzing difficult medical problems and advising physicians on patient diagnosis. Unfortunately, decades of optimism and arduous work have yielded relatively little in the way of practical bedside tools and have led to a justifiable level of skepticism about the role of computers in medical decisionmaking. Nevertheless, considerable progress has been made through the introduction of increasingly powerful models for problem-solving and the inclusion of more complete pathophysiologic data.[5] In addition, a new generation of computer hardware, which utilizes parallel processing to break highly complex problems into their component parts and process them simultaneously at high speed, has permitted the development of software that can evaluate more complex clinical problems based on much larger databases of clinical findings.

The most promising artificial intelligence strategy for medical applications now appears to be the construction of "neural networks." The key to their application in medicine is the development of a model that simulates the thought process of physicians faced with the same problem. Consider, for example, the problem posed by patients with unexplained fever. The programmer constructs a neural network that parallels the decisionmaking process of the physician confronting an unexplained fever, bringing to bear a variety of relevant clinical and demographic information (sex, age, medical history, physical examination, laboratory tests, X-rays, and so on) to arrive at a proposed diagnosis.

The next step in refining the diagnostic accuracy of the neural network is to select a sample of patients with this complaint who have been cared for by expert physicians and for whom there is both an extensive database of clinical findings and a well-established diagnosis. The data from each such case are then used to "train" the network; that is, in those cases in which an accurate diagnosis has been made by the physician but not by the neural network, the program automatically adjusts the weighting of the different parameters to achieve the best correlation with the known diagnosis. By repeating this process for a large number of documented cases, it is possible to optimize the diagnostic performance of the program.

The practicing physician confronted with an actual case of unexplained fever enters the clinical and patient-profile data called for by the program and receives from the computer a response based on the "training" the computer has had. The response could either propose a diagnosis or indicate the need for further tests. Such systems are still in their infancy, and the hard-won success of IBM's "Deep Blue" computer in defeating a human chess player only underlines the difficulty in bringing computers up to a human standard, even in a narrowly circumscribed world like the chess board. Within the next few decades, however, it seems probable that computers will be helping physicians solve increasingly complex clinical puzzles.

Acute myocardial infarction in patients with chest pain can be a difficult diagnosis to make. In a 1991 study, data from 356 patients suspected of having had a myocardial infarction were used to train and test a neural network designed to assist in diagnosis.[6] The network was trained using the clinical findings from one half of the patients, and then tested on its ability to correctly diagnose the other half. The level of accuracy achieved by the network was significantly better than levels previously reported for physicians. A followup study in 1996 yielded similarly encouraging results.[7] Neural networks are also being developed for such applications as predicting the risk of coronary artery bypass grafting, identifying types of brain tumors, predicting the extent of breast cancer invasion, and interpreting electrocardiographic data.

The potential role of computers in "advising" physicians on patient-care decisions will raise a host of thorny questions. Given the extensive memory and problem-solving capability of the computer, what will a doctor still need to know? Should the medical student still be encouraged to accumulate a massive body of facts, or should more attention be given to teaching the student the underlying logic of medical decisionmaking so that he or she can make optimal use of the computer's advice? In my own experience as a supervisor of resident physicians, it seemed that many young physicians failed to make good clinical decisions not for lack of factual knowledge, but because they hadn't been taught the basic steps of medical problem-solving. These skills will continue to be critical even in a highly computerized environment. Even the best-designed programs for clinical problem-solving will not be able to weigh all of the human, environmental, psychological, and social factors, which can only be integrated into the decisionmaking process by an alert and compassionate human practitioner.

And what will be the impact on the doctor-patient relationship when the computer is viewed as the fountain of knowledge? Will patients lose respect for their physician's unaided judgments or will their level of confidence be strengthened by knowing that their physician has such powerful systems close at hand? One potentially valuable result of the increased use of computers in the medical office would be to free up time for thorough, two-way communication between doctor and patient. In theory, there should be more time for physicians to address the emotional toll of disease and to relieve the anxieties of both patient and family by discussing therapeutic options more fully. This potential is not likely to be realized, however, in the new world of managed care. Physicians will be pressed to devote any new-found time they may have to taking on heavier patient loads and speeding more patients through the system.

An interesting area to watch will be the evolution of liability and malpractice law as they deal with these silicon-based consultants. If their advice is bad, how will the culpability be assigned? to the expert panel of physicians who "trained" the program? to the programmers themselves? to the computer manufacturer? And what responsibility will the physician have for ignoring a computed course of action when it is wrong? Is it reasonable to hold physicians to a higher standard of knowledge and intelligence than the computer programs that are advising them? It's only a matter of time before these and other similar issues find their way into the courtroom.

CELL GROWTH STIMULATORS AND TISSUE ENGINEERING

A growing knowledge of the biochemical processes underlying cell growth and regeneration is yielding important new strategies for repairing or replacing damaged tissues and organs. These efforts are to a large extent superseding efforts like the artificial heart, in which organs were replaced with entirely artificial devices. The focus is now on stimulating the body's own repair mechanisms and on propagating replacement tissues outside the body using cell culturing techniques. A wide variety of tissue-engineered products should be ready for general clinical use by the end of this decade.[8]

One early success of this type has been the ability to stimulate the body to regenerate bone tissue lost through disease or accident. The technique relies on naturally occurring substances in the body, called bone morphogenic proteins (BMPs), which stimulate new bone growth by directing immature, unspecialized cells, called stem cells, to grow into bone cells. These substances are responsible for the healing of bone that occurs after a fracture. When they are reproduced in the laboratory in sufficient quantities and introduced at the site of bone loss, they can cause much more substantial regrowth of bone. An early successful application has been in re-growing jaw bone lost through periodontal disease—treatment that previously required bone grafts from other parts of the body. Use of BMPs may help people retain their teeth longer and facilitate tooth implantation into jaw bone when required. BMPs have additional therapeutic potential because they can also stimulate growth and differentiation of other types of cells, like cartilage and ligament cells.

Some other promising applications of laboratory-produced proteins that stimulate cell growth lie in treating spinal damage and hearing loss. Nerve cells have been stubbornly resistant to attempts at inducing regrowth, and, as a result, many victims of traumatic spinal cord injuries have faced the prospect of irreversible paralysis. However, in recent animal experiments it has been shown that when the cut ends of spinal cord cells are bridged by peripheral nerve tissue (from outside the spinal cord) and a nerve growth factor is introduced at the site of the graft, significant regeneration of the spinal cord can occur. In the experiments, regeneration was accompanied by a slight return of function—enough to give the animals a limited ability to stand. There is hope that similar results can eventually be obtained in human patients with acute spinal cord injury—a potential miracle for many.

Restoring hearing loss in the elderly may become possible as researchers work on ways to regrow the tiny hairs that act as sound receptors in the inner ear. When these hairs begin to die off in later life, the resulting hearing loss is permanent, since the damaged cells are not replaced. Palliative treatment has until now relied largely on hearing aids that provide intense overstimulation of the remaining hair cells—generally with less than ideal results. The breakthrough has come from the realization that other mammals have auditory hair cell structures similar to those in humans, which do regenerate.[9] The key questions for investigators become, first, what mechanism is responsible for hair cell regeneration in other animals and, second, whether insights into this mechanism can be applied to the repair of hearing deficits in humans. We now know that activation of a specific signaling pathway within the hair cell, the so-called protein kinase A (PKA) pathway, stimulates auditory hair cell proliferation and that inhibition of PKA blocks this cell growth. Another promising research lead is the discovery that growth factor substances can promote hair cell regeneration in birds; these or analogous agents may ultimately prove effective in humans and thus restore hearing to millions.

Even more exciting than the ability to promote new cell growth in the body is the success researchers have had in growing cell colonies, tissues, and even parts of organs outside the body. Laboratory-grown human skin, for instance, may dramatically improve the prognosis for victims of burns and other trauma and for the common problems of pressure sores in bedridden patients and leg ulcers caused by poor circulation in the elderly. In the past, skin grafting has been hampered by the problem of immunologic rejection. Laboratory-grown human skin avoids this reaction because all the immunogenic components have been left out. One bioengineered skin product currently under development gets its seed cells from the skin removed from newborns during circumcision. These cells are propagated and then disbursed on a sheet of biodegradable fibers, where they multiply and eventually form a new piece of skin. Laboratory-cultured cartilage may be used in a similar way to treat knee injuries. The knee would be repaired by taking tiny quantities of the patient's healthy cartilage cells and propagating them outside the body in quantities sufficient to allow for reconstruction of the injured area. Artificial joint replacement for many knee injuries should no longer be necessary.[10]

Organization of more complex tissue structures is facilitated by the use of fabric "scaffolds" woven out of biodegradable plastics. The scaffolds create the basic structure of the tissue and are seeded with growing populations of the appropriate cell types. The scaffolds induce the cells to act as they would during normal growth processes and help them organize themselves into the appropriate three-dimensional structures—something they don't do if they are simply grown in a petri dish. As the cells propagate and begin to form the new structure, the plastic degrades, and eventually the structure is entirely made up of the new cells. This approach has already been demonstrated in animals, with the successful creation of new heart valves in lambs. It is becoming apparent that cells are surprisingly skilled at reconstituting the structure of their tissue of origin, apparently using the same kinds of intercellular signaling for coordinated growth that they use during embryonic and fetal growth. Although it will be a long time before complex structures can be grown in the laboratory, the near-term prospects look good for growth of simpler structures like blood vessels, heart valves, and urethras.[11]

For organs whose main function is production of needed enzymes and other proteins, an acceptable alternative to replacement of the whole organ may be the implantation of functioning secretory cells taken from donor animals and encapsulated in a material that prevents the body's normal immune reaction against the foreign cells. An artificial pancreas, for instance, is likely to reach the bedside within a decade and transform the treatment of diabetes. Insulin-secreting cells will be harvested from an animal pancreas and then placed in a capsule that allows the insulin to diffuse into the bloodstream in controlled amounts.

MOLECULAR DIAGNOSIS OF GENETIC DISORDERS

The recent advances in molecular biology and experimental genetics have rewritten the textbooks of biology and established the groundwork for an epoch-making change in the diagnosis and treatment of disease. Although it has been established since mid-century that DNA determines the biological characteristics of each individual, it has only been within the past ten years that a new era of molecular medicine has emerged from this knowledge. Molecular medicine will eventually revolutionize every aspect of medical care, but it is first making itself felt by providing a fuller understanding of the causes and underlying defects in various diseases and in the area of genetic screening for hereditary disease.

The DNA in every cell contains the genetic blueprint that determines the structure and function of the entire organism. The "language" of the blueprint resides in the varying sequence of four chemical bases (cytosine, thymine, adenosine, and guanine) along the length of each gene. A full complement of roughly one hundred thousand genes is present in the DNA of every human cell, but only the genes needed for a particular cell's function are active in that cell. Genes exert their effect by providing the instructions for producing specific proteins, the key elements of human cells, tissue, and organs. The instructions are carried from the genes to the ribosomes (the protein-making factories of the cell) with the help of messenger ribonucleic acid (RNA), which is transported out of the nucleus. The messenger RNA in turn directs the arrangement of 20 amino acids into the specified protein. Genetic mutations that induce synthesis of abnormal proteins are now recognized to play a key role in nearly all noninfectious human diseases.

In the research laboratory, we are witnessing worldwide progress toward the Herculean goal of characterizing every one of the genes in the human repertoire. This process is being aided by an imaginative new technology, based on the polymerase chain reaction (PCR), which makes it possible to take a small amount of DNA isolated from a single cell and to replicate it in sufficient quantity to reveal the sequence of bases constituting each gene. Shortly after the turn of the century, this profoundly important effort, known as the Human Genome Project, should have completed the sequencing and location on the chromosomes of every human gene. The knowledge gained from the project will greatly enhance our understanding of the role played by genes in the development of human disease.

To target diseases early in their development, genetic screening for a wide variety of illnesses will soon be a standard part of care— even though treatment and preventive options for those identified as "high-risk" patients may still be limited, as with cancer of the breast. Genetic screening will also yield information on the likelihood of developing other cancers, including prostate and colon cancer, and on a range of other diseases from hypertension to parkinsonism.

Important psychological and ethical issues will arise as screening becomes possible for an ever-larger group of diseases for which no preventive measures are available. For example, patients with a family history of breast cancer face a terrible dilemma in deciding whether it is worse to know or not to know that they themselves are genetically disposed to develop the disease. Two important breast cancer genes have been identified (BRCA1 and BRCA2) that help to identify patients at high risk for developing the disease, but in the absence of reliable preventive measures, prompt diagnosis of the developing disease is the best that can be achieved. In high-risk patients, regular mammography will be started at a younger age than usual and repeated at intervals of perhaps every six months. Some patients may take the extreme step of having a bilateral mastectomy. Unfortunately, even this procedure gives no absolute assurance that cancer will not develop in the tissue left behind.

Physicians and ethicists are equally concerned about the problem of confidentiality, particularly with the growth of large hospital networks, databases of patient records, and the ability to move information readily from one site to another. If genetic information becomes available to employers or insurance companies, serious problems of discrimination will surely arise. In response to these concerns, twelve states have passed laws that would ban insurance companies from using genetic information to deny insurance or to set premiums higher than normal.[12] The Director of the National Center for Genome Research, Dr. Frances S. Collins, summarized the situation this way: "We are all walking around with glitches in our DNA, which place us at risk for something. The information carries the potential to do enormous good for people, in terms of reducing illnesses and suffering. Yet I am deeply concerned that this information can also be turned around to be used against people."[13] Congress, in recognition of this concern, passed legislation in 1996 that forbids group health organizations from denying coverage on the basis of genetic information. A bipartisan effort is under way in Congress to extend this prohibition to all health insurance providers and to further bar insurers from raising premiums based on genetic data. These regulations raise obvious problems for the insurance industry, whose role it is to set premiums by assessing risk, taking into account as much information as possible. A history of previous illnesses, such as heart attack or kidney disease, is routinely used in making such assessments; genetic data—an increasingly reliable indicator of the probability of disease—would be regarded by insurers as a valuable tool.

FIRST SUCCESSES IN MAMMALIAN CLONING

Cloning a human being, long a staple of science fiction, has now been placed within the reach of the possible by the work of a quiet Scottish researcher, Dr. Ian Wilmut, who in early 1997 succeeded in making an exact duplicate of an adult sheep.[14] For a decade or more, scientists have attempted to clone livestock and other mammals but have been frustrated by a seemingly insurmountable hurdle. To clone an adult animal, the nucleus and its DNA from a mature cell has to be transplanted into an egg from which the nucleus has been removed. In a normally fertilized egg, a full spectrum of genes required for all of the differentiated cells of the mature organism is active. But as the embryo grows, and the full complement of DNA is passed on to each new cell, only those genes are active that are needed to fulfill the function of a given type of cell. Most investigators believed that the adult cell with its DNA programmed to fulfill a specific function could not revert to the primitive state that would allow its DNA to instruct the building of a total organism.

Wilmut and his fellow investigators proved that it could, although it reportedly took several decades, a succession of innovative technical maneuvers, and hundreds of implantations to achieve a viable embryo.

The possibility of cloning human beings has understandably

stimulated vigorous debate and federal regulatory action to stifle human cloning research. Many people find the idea of human cloning ethically repugnant, but the arguments about this problem are only beginning. One member of the presidential commission that recommended a ban on human cloning research raised as one troubling problem that "freestanding fertility centers will find themselves called upon by the megalomaniacs of the world to produce for those people the offspring they have always wanted, which is themselves as children."[15] How to tame the new science will become a major social issue as the technology to support human cloning is perfected and as ethically defensible uses of the new technology are proposed.

Of more immediate concern is the fact that all of the research frontiers examined in this chapter will result in new areas of medical diagnosis and therapy for which someone will have to pay. Coming as they do at a time when health care cost containment is an increasing concern, they will exacerbate the already troubling clash between medicine's technological capabilities and society's economic resources to pay for them.

5

Health Care Rationing:
The British Experience

Rationing is a frightening word, particularly in the context of health care. Nevertheless, the "R word" that policymakers dare not utter is slowly coming to the forefront of public consciousness. Bumper stickers proclaiming "Don't Ration My Health Care" provide the most obvious evidence of this new concern. And the worry is not without justification, because the costly medical advances of recent decades are compelling health care providers to consider rationing as a strategy for survival. Needless to say, the word *rationing* itself is rarely uttered publicly by managed care representatives or government officials, but the effect of their actions is the same—the denial of potentially beneficial care to people whose insurance leads them to expect full medical services.

Exactly what form health care rationing in the United States may take in the future is unclear, but one useful predictor is the example of Great Britain. Because of our common heritage in language and culture, along with similar standards of medical training and physician competence, the British experience of the past half-century may hold important lessons for policymakers in this country facing constrained budgets—albeit less severely constrained than in Great Britain.

Some ten years ago, the health care economist Henry Aaron and

I wrote a book on rationing in Britain called *The Painful Prescription: Rationing Hospital Care.*[1] At that time, rationing of health care for the insured was a shocking and unimaginable idea in the United States. When I gave lectures on the British system to business groups and medical organizations like the American Medical Association and American Hospital Association, health professionals and laymen alike were fascinated by the phenomenon of rationing but found it decidedly irrelevant to anything that might happen in the United States. "It can't happen here" was the universal reaction. Today, by contrast, it is practically a given that patients in the United States must be prepared to fight for what they perceive to be their fair share of medical attention.

Although every citizen is nominally entitled to full care, Britain has, in fact, been rationing medical care for decades. Given that the British spend on health care only 37 percent as much per capita as we do in the United States (down from about 50 percent in 1980), British health care providers constantly face tough clinical decisions.[2] In the late 1940s, when the British National Health Service (NHS) was started, experts predicted that after a one-time surge in costs reflecting previously unmet needs, costs would plateau. On the contrary, the rising costs of medical technology have forced the British into a situation where medical resources are increasingly outstripped by demand, and rationing has become a way of life.

The British rationing of care is driven by an overall, nationally determined expenditure ceiling, with primary care physicians paid a fixed annual amount to care for each patient. Hospitals operate on a similarly fixed budget, with occasional extra funds granted for special equipment or programs. To further contain costs, promote equity in care, and allocate limited resources more efficiently, the Thatcher government in 1991 introduced a more market-driven approach. Under this new system, a degree of competition between providers was encouraged, borrowing from the

American idea of "managed competition."[3] The new Labour government has concluded that this approach has been unsuccessful and plans to return to the old system.

One of the most interesting features of rationing in Britain is that many allocation decisions appear irrational if considered on purely medical grounds. Major investments are made in some forms of care that yield only modest medical benefits, while other forms of valuable care are starved for funds. These decisions are apparently driven by nonmedical values and societal pressures. Treatment of the young, for instance, receives far greater support than treatment of the elderly. And a disease like disabling arthritis of the hip, which often forces the patient to struggle with a walker, commands far more resources than angina pectoris (coronary disease), whose symptoms are less visible. Fear of a "dread disease" such as cancer mobilizes a disproportionately large share of resources, even when the particular cancer is incurable. On the whole, physicians and administrators, responding to the fears and prejudices of society, appear to consider many issues other than medical benefits in allocating resources for care.

Confronted with a severe shortage of funds and by conflicting medical and economic imperatives, how do physicians actually interact with their patients? Doctors in Britain, it has been said, ration "by rationalization" in order to avoid actually saying no. They have made denial of care palatable to themselves as well as to patients by adopting an informal consensus on acceptable thresholds for intervention far higher than any medically desirable level. For example, patients with coronary artery disease are not recommended for angioplasty until their pain is far more severe than would mandate treatment by even the most conservative physicians in the United States.

Many British doctors are well aware that they are acting as society's agents in the rationing process. One highly regarded authority spoke of the process as follows:

The sense that I have is that there are many situations where resources are sufficiently short so that there must be decisions made as
to who is treated. Given that circumstance, the physician, in order
to live with himself and to sleep well at night, has to look at the
arguments for not treating a patient. And there are always some—
social, medical, whatever. In many instances he heightens, sharpens,
or brings into focus the negative component in order to make himself and the patient comfortable about not going forward.[4]

Although most British doctors would like to deploy more resources than are now available, they seem to recognize that the
national exchequer is not large enough to provide all the possible
benefits of an ever-expanding arsenal of medical interventions. Intensive care is a good example. In a major London teaching hospital
with nearly a thousand beds, there are only ten intensive care beds,
about one-tenth the number there would be in a similar American
hospital. The physician in charge of intensive care, responding to
a question about whether his unit should be expanded, summed
up his views like this: "No. It has to be appropriate to the sur-
roundings. Now, what we have by your standards is way short of
the mark. It would be too small in America, but if you took this
unit and put it down in the middle of Sri Lanka or India, it would
stick out like a sore thumb. It would be an obscene waste of
money."[5]

British physicians are often spared having to deny treatment explicitly by the long waiting lists most patients endure before being
accepted for noncritical procedures. Waits of weeks or months for
elective surgery discourage many patients from opting for care to
which they are entitled. Requiring patients in need of a specialist's
care to first schedule an appointment with a primary care physician
has a similar inhibitory effect. Although neither of these strategies
involves explicit denial of services, patients are nevertheless aware
that their access to medical services is being reduced. Only in the
last several years has the word *rationing* begun to appear in British
discussions on resource allocation.

A 1995 survey of regional health authorities revealed that restrictions on care were no longer limited to treatments of dubious
value but also to preventive services such as ultrasound tests in
pregnancy and screening tests for osteoporosis, aortic aneurysm,
and colorectal cancers, as well as to demonstrably effective treatments such as surgery for varicose veins and various therapies for
infertility. A prominent commentator noted: "Rationing is as old
as the NHS. Initially it was implicitly applied (queues, waiting lists,
waiting times), but has gradually become more explicit: diabetics
refused renal dialysis, the elderly denied intensive care, people with
alcoholism refused liver transplants."[6] The recently elected Labour
government campaigned on a promise of infusing enough new
money into the NHS to reduce substantially the need for rationing
of any kind, but it remains to be seen if such promises can with-
stand the pressure of fiscal reality.

Even in a nominally egalitarian system, such as the British
one, the wealthy and well-informed have learned how to escape
most of the system's budget constraints. They circumvent the long
queues for non-emergency surgery through the purchase of private
insurance that covers such procedures as hip replacement or hernia
repair, which are typically performed by leading surgeons within
a few days or weeks. If denied complex care that is available only
within sophisticated National Health Care hospitals, affluent and
influential British patients simply won't take no for an answer.
They use a variety of techniques to circumvent the system, including phone calls to influential friends. Hip replacement surgeries are
difficult to obtain at any age, but not long ago one was carried out
on a very lucky 93-year-old—the Queen Mother.

EXPERIENCES IN OTHER EUROPEAN NATIONS

Although the United States has been struggling with rapidly rising
health care costs for more than a decade, only in the last several
years have spiraling costs imperiled the generous government-

sponsored health plans in many European countries. For the first time, health care costs throughout western Europe are being viewed as a serious problem requiring effective cost-containment measures. In France and Germany, as in England, the root cause of the problem is identified as system inefficiency and wasteful use of the system by physicians and patients. The countermeasures being proposed are largely familiar ones: bringing into play market forces and the cost-saving incentives of managed care. Increased computerization of health care records is also being touted as a way to monitor and rein in costs.

In France, the health system has been in the red every year since 1990, with deficits reaching $6.5 billion to $8 billion annually, and the government is coming under increasing pressure to act. In a tactic familiar to American managed care patients, freedom to bypass the general practitioner and make direct contact with a specialist is being eliminated. The government has traditionally paid 65 percent of the cost of drugs; in an attempt to ease this burden, the French premier in 1996 ordered pharmaceutical companies to pay $500 million as a "contribution" to the health insurance fund because they have profited so handsomely from the government's subsidy. In some desperation, the French government also ordered physicians to slow the rise in total expenditures to 2.1 percent per year, only to find that the fiscal river had already overflowed its banks by 6.1 percent in the first half of the year. Said one French physician: "I wonder how long patients will continue to trust doctors they know have a financial interest in saving money."[7] The director of the French National Fund for Sickness Insurance recently remarked: "The main hope is to be able to make sufficient savings by making care more efficient, while not reducing benefits, but our plan could be too little too late"—an unusually honest evaluation of a strategy that will almost certainly prove inadequate to the task at hand.

In Germany, the move toward managed care is rapid. "Our sys-

tem is like a big HMO," said Dr. Gunnar Griesewell of the German
Health Ministry in Bonn. The pressure on doctors is becoming
intense, and oversubscribing is necessitating cuts in payments to
physicians. In the Netherlands, there is a move toward eliminating
funding for therapies that have not been conclusively proven effective through rigorous outcome studies. That could result in the
exclusion of over half of the therapies currently provided, and the
welter of problems surrounding the interpretation of outcome
studies will pose a formidable obstacle to implementation.

THE CANADIAN SYSTEM

In Canada, which has a single-payer national health insurance program, the problem of rising costs is said to be appreciably eased
by the lower administrative costs of a unified system. Because these
costs are claimed to be substantially lower than in the United States,
many observers have urged moving the United States to a centralized system.[8] In fact, reliable analysts have concluded that administrative costs in the United States are no higher than those in
Canada once adjustments are made for differences in cost accounting practices.[9]

Regardless of whether Canada has a more efficient system, it
appears to be beleaguered by troubles that have eroded much of
the public's confidence in its medical care. Canada is confronting
the same problems as other countries plagued by the rise in health
care costs. Cuts in budgets have led to hospital consolidation, reduced nursing staff, and long waiting times for non-emergency
surgery. Patients who have seen a primary care physician and require consultation with a specialist typically have to wait eight
weeks for an appointment. A severe shortage of staffing and equipment, such as MRIs, CT scanners, and open-heart surgical units,
appears to be a major cause of the reduced quality of care.

These problems have contributed to a substantial number of

dissatisfied physicians leaving Canada each year—2,500 out of 55,000 between 1991 and 1994.[10] Patients who cannot get the high-tech care they want find their way to U.S. hospitals. A new commercial organization in Canada now buys, at discounted prices, the right to advanced medical procedures at high-quality institutions in the United States. These rights are then resold to Canadian insurance companies that write policies for travelers. The negative reports from Canada may be exaggerated, but the evidence at hand offers little reason to believe that Canada has solved the problem of controlling costs while sustaining high-quality care.

6

Managed Care and Rationing

in the United States

The early years of managed care in the United States, led by in-
novators like the Kaiser Permanente system in California, were
viewed by almost all observers as showing tremendous promise
for curtailing costs without jeopardizing quality of care. From the
1950s until the early 1980s, managed care providers (almost ex-
clusively HMOs) supplied services at a cost much lower than the
fee-for-service sector while imposing little or no rationing. The
reason was simple: for decades HMOs used some 30 percent fewer
hospital days per enrollee than did the fee-for-service sector.[1] The
lower rate of use was achieved by eliminating days of hospitalization that offered negligible benefit to the patient and thus permitted savings with little or no sacrifice of quality. A classic study
has shown that no other factor in the managed care system has
contributed appreciably to its cost advantage.[2] In particular, the
study found no evidence that the highly touted advantage of a
health maintenance approach, that is, an emphasis on preventive
medicine and coordinated care, had any appreciable effect on the
health of enrollees or on costs.

Although the level of HMO premiums and expenditures was below that of the fee-for-service sector, the *rate of increase* in costs in
HMOs was indistinguishable from that in the fee-for-service sec-

tor.³ Such a parallel rise was inevitable if HMOs were to provide patients with full access to the endless stream of expensive new technology. And as the U.S. health care system as a whole has cut back on days of hospitalization, the early cost advantage of HMOs has been largely eliminated. To remain competitive, managed care providers have begun to institute policies that hold down costs by limiting the quantity and, to some extent, the quality of the care provided. Insured Americans still find it hard to believe that they might be denied any potentially useful care. But because other strategies for achieving cost containment in the health care system have already been largely exhausted, effective cost containment will undoubtedly require that some beneficial services be denied to some patients.

A flurry of recent regulatory activity reflects a sudden public and political awareness of this disturbing situation, but its inevitable development has been obvious for at least a decade. My 1988 editorial on the subject in the *Wall Street Journal* was considered to be unduly pessimistic at the time, but ten years later its predictions seem fairly close to the mark:

At least for a time, HMOs will probably be able to compete by reducing service without the patient's knowledge. Most patients will not be aware of an expensive test forgone or a consultation not provided—omissions that can readily escape detection if they are limited in scope. But when the outer bounds of this strategy have been reached, HMOs almost certainly will become more forthright about what they are offering. To meet the test of the marketplace, they are likely to openly differentiate themselves according to price, range of services, and quality. In the highly competitive marketplace that is now evolving, many health maintenance organizations may well be impelled to change their style from lean to mean. But most important, it now seems clear that employers and governments must give up their fantasy that HMOs have some magic that can provide a painless path to fiscal salvation.⁴

All of the major players in the U.S. health care delivery system find themselves under mounting pressure to offer services at the lowest possible cost. Hospitals threatened by large deficits and potential bankruptcy are seeking to preserve or increase market share. But as the pool of patients needing hospitalization shrinks, contract negotiations with managed care organizations are becoming cutthroat. The managed care organizations, in turn, are under pressure from employers to lower premiums by clamping down on hospital and physician costs. They are typically concerned about controlling the "loss ratio," the figure that represents how much of their income must actually be spent on patient care. Physicians and other health professionals are at the center of the struggle, caught between their desire to offer the best possible care for their patients and their need to survive in the harsh new medical marketplace, where jobs are scarce and everyone is expendable.

Although the health care rationing that arises from these pressures can take many guises, the two major types of rationing already emerging are (1) limiting the availability of very expensive procedures such as bone marrow transplantation and (2) reducing the general level of care for common diseases that don't involve single big-ticket procedures (but have high costs in the aggregate). To achieve these ends, the incentives offered to physicians in the managed care sector are almost diametrically opposite from what they were when physicians acted as independent providers.

As an individual practitioner, the physician in a fee-for-service environment had every reason to do the best for the insured patient regardless of cost. More visits or more lab tests meant little additional expense to the patient because the patient's insurance was picking up the tab. This indifference to cost naturally made it too easy for physicians to err on the side of excess. Their motivation was not simply to safeguard their patients' health but also to protect themselves against malpractice suits through the practice of so-called defensive medicine. Because some physicians had a financial stake in the laboratory and imaging facilities they used, there was a further incentive to do more than was medically justified.

Managed care has gone a long way toward shifting the balance of the physician's priorities. An important role of the managed care physician is now to identify and eliminate demonstrably useless care. Indeed, under increasing economic pressure, the physician is expected to discourage or deny access to care that is seen as only marginally useful. As a result, the best interest of the patient is no longer the physician's exclusive concern in deciding on a course of treatment. A more realistic guiding principle is now to maximize the therapeutic benefits within given budgetary constraints.

EARLY SYMPTOMS OF RATIONING

Out of the altered realities of managed care are growing a variety of impediments to obtaining medical care. In New York State, for instance, investigators cited 13 of 18 HMOs for substandard care because patients had difficulty getting appointments to see a physician.[5] At one HMO in Manhattan, 69 percent of obstetricians and 40 percent of pediatricians could not provide appointments for routine examinations. Although hard data like this are still difficult to come by, some common symptoms of managed care's concern for the bottom line are becoming clear:

- long delays in obtaining appointments and long waits in the doctor's office are discouraging use of services and reducing quality of care
- physicians spending unduly brief amounts of time with each patient
- effective, state-of-the-art procedures being declared "experimental" (and therefore not covered by the plan) until long after they have been widely accepted by experts in the medical community

- physicians being required to obtain approval for many treatments from a non-physician, particularly for expensive procedures

- patients finding that certain treatments are excluded from coverage, based on the fine print in their contracts, and that arbitration of disputes about covered services is under the control of the managed care provider

- physicians being encouraged to consult with other physicians by phone, without the consultant seeing the patient

- patients having trouble obtaining reimbursement for emergency care if it is provided at a hospital that is not part of the patient's managed care network

- severe restrictions on mental health services, especially through rules limiting the number of psychotherapy sessions covered and through discouraging use of psychotherapy in combination with drug therapy. By these means, managed care programs for mental health have reportedly cut their expenditures by some 30 percent.[6]

Although the effects of these practices on clinical outcomes have been for the most part unquantified, their effects on patients' *perceptions* about quality of care are beginning to be measured, and the results are not reassuring. In late 1997 the results of a survey undertaken by researchers at Harvard University and the Kaiser Family Foundation revealed a widespread lack of confidence in the managed care system:

- Sixty percent of respondents said managed care has reduced the amount of time doctors spend with patients and made it harder for patients to see specialists.

- Fifty-five percent of those surveyed indicated concern that if they become ill, their managed care provider will be more interested in saving money than in providing optimal care.

- While 76 percent of respondents with traditional fee-for-service insurance gave their plans a grade of A or B, only 66 percent of respondents with managed care plans did so. Ten percent of respondents in managed care gave grades of D or E to their plans, compared to only 4 percent of respondents with fee-for-service plans.

- Only 28 percent of those surveyed felt that managed care has helped keep medical costs down.

Drew Altman, president of the Kaiser Family Foundation (an independent national health care philanthropy not associated with the Kaiser Permanente HMO) summarized the results by saying that "managed care is winning in the health care marketplace, but is in danger of losing the battle for public opinion."[7]

Local and national regulations to protect patients against denial of care are already being enacted. In fact Congress and state legislatures around the country are clogged with pending bills aimed at making it more difficult for managed care organizations to deny care: over one thousand such bills have been introduced in 39 states, and approximately one hundred have been introduced in Congress.[8] In California, where state agencies registered more than two thousand complaints about HMOs in 1996, roughly a hundred separate pieces of regulatory legislation were under consideration in late 1997.

Some of these state and federal initiatives focus on forcing managed care plans to give patients more information about covered and excluded services. Some attempt to give patients a more convenient avenue of redress when they feel that services are being unfairly denied, and some forbid financial rewards to doctors for denying care. Others mandate direct access to gynecologists for female patients and require coverage of out-of-network emergency room visits, even if it turns out that the visit was not a medical necessity. But so far the most active regulatory areas have been in restoring to physicians their authority in determining length of hospitalization (most notably for childbirth and mastectomy) and their freedom to communicate with patients about all treatment options without fear of reprisal. In the absence of a coordinated and comprehensive strategy for regulation of the managed care industry, however, managed care organizations will engage in a cat-and-mouse game with regulatory authorities, in which effective regulatory action on one front simply leads to the development of new cost-cutting strategies on another.

Physician Gag Rules Confidentiality clauses, or "gag rules," have been included in many contracts between managed care providers and physicians, with the goal of preventing physicians from sharing information with patients that might lead to patient dissatisfaction with the plan. Physicians have been forbidden to talk with patients about treatment plans without administrative authorization. They have also been barred from revealing the practice guidelines that underlie their decisions or disclosing any financial incentives in their contracts to keep expenditures under specified amounts.

Physicians and patients alike have complained that the doctor-patient relationship is seriously compromised by such restrictions. Recently, contractual limitations on discussion of treatment options have been disallowed by a directive from both the federal government and by the trade association of private managed care organizations. However, the effectiveness of such regulatory efforts is uncertain, and Congress is already drafting legislation to bolster them. In an attempt to stay a step ahead of the regulators, the American Association of Health Plans has also instructed its member organizations not to prevent doctors from revealing the basis of their remuneration to patients. For example, physicians should be free to acknowledge that they are financially rewarded for controlling costs and that they are penalized for spending too much. How faithfully managed care organizations will protect physicians' rights in this area is uncertain. Again, it may well take the pressure of federal legislation to assure widespread compliance.

Limiting Specialized Care   As managed care organizations reduce their pool of specialists to keep costs down, referrals for specialized care are becoming less common. As a result, many well-trained specialists in areas like gastroenterology, cardiology, and nephrology are being forced to shift to family practice, pediatrics, and general internal medicine. Consequently, generalist physicians are being called on to accept responsibility for increasingly complex and difficult cases. A similar shift is taking place within the specialties themselves. A general orthopedist, for example, may be given responsibility for complex hand surgery, even though the best care requires a subspecialist whose practice is limited to such surgery.

Although it is generally agreed that specialists can make a significant clinical difference in the handling of difficult and unusual cases, there is less consensus on the usefulness of specialists in the management of relatively common disorders like heart attack. However, a recent study showed that heart attack victims fared significantly better under the care of a cardiologist rather than a primary care physician.[9] The cardiologists' patients were 12 percent less likely to die in the first year than were patients cared for by generalists. The better outcomes were achieved in part through more extensive use of specialized therapeutic procedures and drugs. To eliminate the difference in death rate, it would be necessary to provide cardiologists for all heart attack patients—a change that would wreak havoc with plans to reduce numbers of specialists. It remains to be seen whether specialists in other areas can muster similar evidence of improved outcomes. So far, managed care providers have been understandably reticent about explaining how and why they reach the decisions they do concerning levels of specialty staffing.

Savings in Routine Hospital Care   Many of the cost-saving strategies instituted by managed care organizations put particular pressure on hospitals to control the costs of inpatient stays. As a result, we are likely to see a variety of cost-cutting measures in hospitals, some of which affect previously sacrosanct aspects of modern hospital care:

· Use of the postoperative recovery room, a valuable
  safety environment for patients during a risky period,
  will be less common, and more patients will be sent
  directly from the surgical suite to the hospital floor.

· Following the lead of Great Britain, the number of intensive care beds will be reduced, and the depth of
  staffing in such units as well as the investment in new
  equipment will be cut back.

· Hospital stays will be shortened even beyond the reductions that have already taken place, with a probable increase in post-discharge complications.

· There will be an ongoing erosion of staffing by registered nurses. Highly paid senior nurses will be especially attractive layoff targets and will be replaced in
  many cases by relatively untrained nurse's aides.
  Chronic understaffing will lead to longer response
  times in reacting to patient distress and medical emergencies. Cuts in personnel other than nurses will de-
  grade quality of care in departments such as X-ray,
  dietary services, and physiotherapy.

· Hospitals will substitute cheaper, lower-quality versions of commonly used supplies like injectable dyes for imaging.

· University-affiliated hospitals in academic medical centers will curtail their teaching programs on hospital wards because staff time will be too limited for the kind of in-depth discussions that are essential to high-quality training.

· Large new equipment purchases will be subject to rigorous scrutiny. As a result, high-technology equipment manufacturers will think long and hard before making the enormous investment in research and development required for a major new device. (Reconditioned, second-hand equipment is becoming a financially attractive alternative to new equipment purchases in hospitals.)

SACRIFICING THE HUMANITY IN PATIENT CARE

This discussion of the technical and economic aspects of health care rationing has given short shrift to the human pain and suffering that represent the hidden cost of rationing. I leave it to others to explore this human dimension in detail, but it is clear that the pressures of cost containment are forcing caregivers to spend less time talking (and listening) to patients and helping them through the anxieties and fears of illness.

I had a deeply painful experience with a member of my own family that brought this issue home to me. In late 1994, my forty-year-old son was diagnosed with inoperable lung cancer. During his courageous battle with that disease, he wrote an article for the *Boston Globe Magazine* about what it was like to be a seriously ill patient in a large metropolitan hospital.[10] In particular, he described how much comfort he derived from the many seemingly minor ways in which his physicians and other caregivers reached out to him as a human being, sometimes with just a reassuring word or a touch. But he also expressed a deep unease about the future of such humanely administered care in an era of ever tighter cost accountability. His words speak for themselves.

Until last fall, I had spent a considerable part of my career as a health-care lawyer, first in the state government and then in the private sector. I came to know a lot about health care policy and management, government regulations and contracts. But I knew little about the delivery of care. All that changed on November 7, 1994, when at age 40 I was diagnosed with advanced lung cancer. In the months following, I was subjected to chemotherapy, radiation, surgery, and news of all kinds, most of it bad. It has been a harrowing experience for me and for my family. And yet, the ordeal has been punctuated by moments of exquisite compassion. I have been the recipient of an extraordinary array of human and humane responses to my plight. These acts of kindness—the simple human touch from my care-givers—have made the unbearable bearable. . . .

In my new role as patient, I have learned that medicine is not merely about performing tests or surgeries, or administering drugs. These functions, important as they are, are just the beginning. For as skilled and knowledgeable as my caregivers are, what matters most is that they have empathized with me in a way that gives me hope and makes me feel like a human being, not just an illness. Again and again, I have been touched by the smallest kind gestures—a squeeze of my hand, a gentle touch, a reassuring word. In some ways, these quiet acts of humanity have felt more healing than the high-dose radiation and chemotherapy that hold the hope of a cure.

I deeply appreciate the care I have had as a patient. But I can't help wondering why I have had such a heartening experience. Is it attributable to the exceptional quality of care and caring delivered at Massachusetts General Hospital? Is it due to the particular caregivers that I happened to meet? Or have I benefited in some way from my family's medical connections, since my father and brother were trained in Boston academic institutions and have ties to senior MGH physicians? Perhaps my experience has not been the result of happenstance or special relationships but of a health-care environment that still places the patient ahead of the bottom line.

If so, for how long will such a compassionate approach endure? Medicaid and Medicare cuts, both present and future, will have devastating effects on hospital care. Managed care is already making its mark in Massachusetts, and it will only accelerate implementation of its cardinal principles: efficiency, conservation of time and resources, and budget cuts. And now, for-profit insurers and large national hospital chains are trying to penetrate Massachusetts for the first time. In such a cost-conscious world, with its inevitable reductions in staff and morale, can any hospital continue to nurture those precious moments of engagement between patient and caregiver that provide hope to the patient and vital support to the healing process?

Time—in short supply with managed care physicians and nurses—is a prerequisite for real engagement between caregiver and patient. Even the most compassionate caregivers cannot use their healing gifts if they don't have the time to do so. A friend who worked at the National Cancer Institute, in Maryland, quoted his mentor as saying that when physicians give bad news to a patient, they must give that person more of their time—to explain, to answer questions, and provide comfort.

Time alone is not enough, however. Caregivers need to be trained and encouraged to engage with their patients. My understanding is that medical-school training now emphasizes to a greater degree the importance of the physician-patient relationship, a bond that ultimately reaffirms the humanity of both. As an eminent Harvard Medical School professor, himself a cancer patient, once taught: "The secret of the care of the patient is caring for the patient."

This experience has made me wonder whether my son is among the last beneficiaries of such humane care and whether it can survive the crushing pressures on hospitals and physicians in the coming decades. What is especially disturbing about this development is that shortchanging the humane component of hospital care yields at best a one-time reduction in level of spending on personnel. It doesn't in any way address the long-term problem of escalating expenditures on technology; it simply undermines a key component of care.

RATIONING TARGETED AT THE ELDERLY AND THE TERMINALLY ILL

The rationing phenomena that we have looked at so far affect patients across the board. However, it seems likely that patients who are very old or who appear to be terminally ill will be especially vulnerable to the kinds of corner-cutting and denial of services that we have discussed. In Great Britain it is clear that the elderly are viewed as having enjoyed their fair share of life and are given markedly less aggressive care for life-threatening illnesses. Admission to the hospital is discouraged, indeed restricted, and intensive care is sharply limited. Similar unwritten policies will almost certainly play a growing role in the U.S. health care system, and indeed one leading medical ethicist has proposed elimination of life-extending care for most people over the age of 75.

This mode of rationing has obvious appeal to the young. But, aside from the many ethical concerns it raises, it probably would make only a modest contribution to slowing the rise in costs of medical care. Currently, people aged 75 or older constitute less than 6 percent of the United States population. However, because per capita medical costs for the very old run about three to seven times the national average, those costs do account for about one-fifth of annual health care spending. Still, abruptly eliminating a third of the services used by this group—a truly ambitious goal, because no one has proposed denying lifesaving care to otherwise healthy old people—would produce a one-time reduction of only a few percent in total health care expenditures.[11]

There will also be pressure to limit major, life-extending interventions for those patients who are judged to be terminally ill. Such interventions are an attractive target for cutbacks, not least because care in the last year of life consumes some 10 to 12 percent of the nation's health care dollars.[12] Moreover, the benefits of aggressive care at the end of life are not always clear and may add needlessly to the patient's suffering.

It is doubtful, however, that any significant long-term savings can be accomplished by restricting access to aggressive measures at the end of life. While it is easy to calculate in retrospect how much money would have been saved if aggressive care had not been provided for the terminally ill, it is considerably more difficult prospectively to distinguish those patients who are indeed terminal from those who might still benefit from aggressive care. Various studies have calculated only modest savings, ranging from zero to 10 percent of current expenditures. The larger the study and the longer the period of observation, the smaller the observed savings. Better designed and controlled experiments will be needed to settle this question.

BRINGING RATIONING INTO THE OPEN

Given the virtual certainty of a mounting imperative to ration care, we will soon need to decide how we will allocate this country's enormous but not inexhaustible health care resources. "Muddling through" in the British way, that is, making rationing decisions only in a tacit and ad hoc manner, may prove to be the only practical and politically acceptable approach. But the American public's growing awareness of the health care they are getting—and not getting—suggests that a strategy based on unspoken understandings and deliberate euphemisms may not be enough. The next chapter addresses the difficult question of how we might tackle the problems of resource allocation in a more open and logically defensible way. There will be no easy answers, but failure to take on this challenge can only lead to continued turmoil in the health care system as insured patients—taking on faith that everything possible is being done for them—discover to their consternation that the rules of the game have changed.

7

A large proportion of medical resources is allocated through the thousands of minor decisions physicians and other caregivers make each day, typically without seriously or systematically weighing the costs of care against potential benefits. And there is probably no practical way to oversee these myriad decisions or to imbue them with a more rigorous logic. On the other hand, roughly half of acute care expenditures are attributable to major, resource-intensive interventions, such as heart surgery, organ transplantation, and admittance to intensive care units.[1] And there may be hope that at least the decisions to initiate or forgo these expensive interventions can be subjected to some form of structured analysis. Certainly if federal and local regulations begin forcing managed care providers to reveal the basis of their patient care decisions, there will be a growing need to justify them in an organized way.

Oregon is the first and so far the only state to implement a systematic and explicit approach to rationing expensive medical interventions. Although there are serious defects in the Oregon program, the state deserves credit for its pioneering efforts to de-mystify the allocation of limited medical resources. The plan relies on a budget constraint that fixes the amount of money available for state-funded care and then ranks the efficacy of specific disease-treatment pairs (e.g., hip replacement for severe arthritis, coronary bypass surgery for heart attack). Interventions that fall above a cut-off point determined by the available funds are made available to all. Those that fall below the cutoff line are not funded for any patients, regardless of the improvement that might be expected in individual cases.

The plan raises three troublesome issues. First, because it affects only Medicaid patients, those on limited incomes, it raises serious questions of fairness. Second, in their efforts to reduce the number of disease entities to a manageable size, the Oregon regulators have lumped together diseases of very different character and severity. Third, and most problematic of all, is the fact that the Oregon plan nearly always assigns only a single benefit value to each disease-treatment pair, even though the same treatment for a given disease can provide widely varying medical benefits depending on the patient: the severity of the disease, the patient's age, and other concurrent diseases all affect the outcome. Ranking disease-treatment pairs for their clinical efficacy makes little sense when the end results are so dissimilar in different patients.

Consider, for example, a stricture of the esophagus that causes obstruction and difficulty in swallowing. Depending on the severity, which can vary widely, this condition may require totally different interventions. Mild narrowing can often be managed simply with medication and a change in diet. More severe narrowing requires mechanical techniques that stretch the esophagus. Still more severe disease demands surgery. If corrective surgery fails, it may be necessary to replace the esophagus by a loop of bowel—a risky procedure, particularly in patients with lung or heart disease. In this case neither the costs of intervention nor the expected benefit to patients can be reduced to any simple formula. The Oregon plan provides support for surgical treatment of esophageal stricture, even though in many patients surgical intervention would constitute a serious misallocation of funds.

Surgery for colon cancer also defies any simple effort at ranking the usefulness of clinical interventions. If the tumor is limited to the lining of the bowel, 80 to 90 percent of patients will survive surgery for ten years or more. If the cancer has penetrated the bowel wall, survival rate drops substantially, and with involvement of the adjacent lymph nodes, it falls to about one-third. If the cancer has migrated to other parts of the body, surgery is of no value except to relieve obstruction of the bowel. The Oregon plan provides funding for all colon cancer surgery, even for those patients with little or no prospect of recovery.

As these examples indicate, classifying all instances of a clinical condition and an associated therapy under one ranking, and determining whether to pay for the therapy on the basis of this single ranking, grossly oversimplifies clinical outcomes. A rationing system that cannot distinguish between a mild and a severe form of a disease or between the prognosis for that disease in an otherwise healthy patient and in a patient with a concurrent complicating disease is a crude system indeed. If medical care is to be rationed in a sensible way, this all-or-nothing approach must be refined. The Oregon approach, although well-intentioned, will inevitably lead to a misallocation of resources; that is, available resources will not be used by the Oregon system in a way that maximizes medical benefits on a per-dollar basis.

EQUALIZING THE BENEFITS OF MEDICAL INTERVENTIONS AT THE MARGIN

In principle there is a more equitable way to set limits on the use of medical interventions, and it might open the way for a more medically and ethically defensible system of rationing in the future. The goal is to avoid the complete elimination of particular expensive medical interventions, but instead to limit the application of all expensive interventions to those patients most likely to benefit.

The strategy is designed to ensure that the last dollar spent on each type of expensive technology yields roughly equivalent benefits. This is a principle familiar from microeconomics, but it has not previously been applied to health care resources.

EXPECTED BENEFIT AND THE BENEFITS CURVE

To ensure that the last dollar spent on each different technology will indeed yield a similar benefit requires a comparison of the "expected benefit" in different patients. *Expected benefit*, a term drawn from standard economics, is defined as the probability of an intervention succeeding, multiplied by the value to the patient of that intervention (measured in terms of pain reduction, increased mobility, extension of life, etc.). This formulation translates into the simple equation $EB = P \times B$, where EB is the expected benefit, P the probability of success and B the degree of benefit that can be anticipated. When either the probability of success or the degree of benefit goes up, the expected benefit rises. When either goes down, the expected benefit falls.

Because different patients suffering from the same disease often experience different degrees and complications of the illness, the expected benefit of an intervention can range from life-saving to negligible. This variation can be depicted graphically in a "benefits curve" by plotting the values for expected benefit through a sequence of patient groups ranging from the most promising to the least promising candidates. Figure 1 represents a hypothetical benefits curve showing the variation in expected benefits for a group of patients receiving a particular therapy for a given disease. Some patients (plotted on the left) benefit substantially from treatment and some (the right side of the curve) benefit only marginally.

Different medical interventions obviously have very different benefits curves. In trying to allocate limited resources to the different interventions in a way that maximizes benefits, the task is

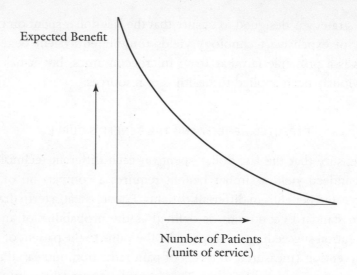

FIGURE 1.   A hypothetical benefits curve. Expected benefit is plotted
on the vertical axis and is calculated by multiplying the probability of
an intervention having a favorable effect by the magnitude of the benefit. Some patients (plotted on the left) stand to benefit substantially
from treatment, while others will probably benefit only marginally
(plotted on the right). Benefits curves may have very different shapes
depending on the particular condition and intervention.

to find the cutoff point on all of the benefits curves where the
benefits are roughly equal and all of the dollars available under a
given budget constraint have been spent. In the real world, it would
not be necessary to look closely at the patient groups at the top of
the curve (those whose chances of substantial improvement are
great), but only to focus at the bottom of the curve, that 10 to 15
percent of patients whose potential benefit from the intervention
is smallest and who therefore will be the prime targets for reallo-
cation of resources.

This procedure for comparing expected benefits across a range
of technologies works well if each technology costs roughly the
same amount per patient. However, since this is typically not true,
a more useful point of comparison is the *expected benefit per dollar*. That

is, the expected benefit calculation must in turn be divided by the cost of the intervention in order to arrive at a ratio of benefits per dollar. Even an intervention with a high expected benefit may have a relatively low ratio of benefit per dollar if it is very expensive. For example, a $200,000 heart transplant with a high expected benefit for a particular patient may have a lower benefits-per-dollar quotient than a $50,000 hip replacement for a patient with a much lower expected benefit.

A homely example of the way in which expected benefits per dollar can be equalized for different types of expenditures can be drawn from household budget planning. Let us assume that a family whose income is fixed and fully committed to a variety of ordinary household expenditures needs to buy a car. The old one is on its last legs, and transportation is required to get family members to work. Because they have no savings, they can buy the car only by shifting money from other household expenditures. Possible targets for cuts include all categories of expenditure—utilities, food, clothing, cleaning, insurance, entertainment, saving for college, medical care. Under these circumstances, the necessary economies can probably better be achieved by trimming several categories of consumption than by eliminating any single category entirely. The family might decide to lower the thermostat in winter, but not go without heat altogether, and to reduce the number of movie outings, but not eliminate moviegoing altogether. How much each area is cut back depends on the value the family places on it, its relative expense, and the severity of the budget constraint. The goal, as we have said, is to assure that the last dollar spent in each area of the household budget yields roughly equivalent benefits. If it doesn't, then the money must be shifted from an area of low benefit to an area of higher benefit in order to get the greatest value from the available dollars.

Consider now an analogous medical situation in which a managed care organization has a fixed pool of money available for the year to cover every component of care for each enrolled patient. Suddenly a new technology becomes available, perhaps an expensive new anticancer drug that will extend the life of afflicted patients for 10 or 15 years. How might a managed care group decide what to do? Like the family trying to finance car payments, it will need to trim those expenditures that are producing the least benefit per dollar if it is to accommodate the new, high-value technology. More specifically, it must confront the difficult task of identifying and excluding from other treatments those candidates for treatment who can be expected to benefit least. Such patients may, for example, have complicating illnesses and thus have a poorer prospect of recovery from major surgery. Dollars must then be shifted away from these patients for whom the promise of benefit is small, leaving intact the funding of the procedures for those patients who have the prospect of more substantial gains. Like the belt-tightening family, the managed care group should be able to maximize benefits by being more stringent across all areas of expenditure, rather than by eliminating any areas entirely.

Even under a fixed budget, new technology can be accommodated and aggregate medical benefits can actually increase if low-benefit uses of expensive care are stripped away and the dollars applied to high-benefit uses of the new technology.

Needless to say, there are some stumbling blocks in implementing this sort of approach. One is the problem of quantifying an expected benefit. This requires, first of all, that physicians be prepared to assign probabilities to possible outcomes. Although physicians do this all the time in their daily decisionmaking, they may be loath to make the process more formal or explicit. Obviously, some predictions about the chance of successful outcomes are rough approximations at best, but the growing literature of well-controlled outcome studies in different patient populations should help refine these predictions in the coming years.

An even more formidable obstacle is the need to quantify and compare the values of the outcomes themselves. Only by assigning some sort of quantitative value to the desired medical outcomes is it possible to arrive at values for expected benefits that can be weighed against each other. But where does one begin? Does a reduction in cardiac pain from severe to mild score higher than restoration of a normal range of motion in a disabled hip? Does relief of the embarrassment caused by severe acne scars outrank a modest improvement in hearing? Is an extension of life by six months more beneficial than restoring the ability to enjoy a normal sex life?

Physicians may have their own ideas about how these benefits compare, but these judgments are ultimately not scientific ones. And for this reason, it may be best to consider a means whereby the community at large can be involved in assigning comparative values to at least the general classes of medical outcomes. In fact, the early Seattle experience with rationing of kidney dialysis, described in chapter 1, established a precedent for involving members of the community in handling the subjective aspects of rationing decisions. Although the practical challenges of convening community panels to quantify the value of medical outcomes may make them unworkable, some means of characterizing the community's outlook on treatment priorities must be found.

As a result of all these difficulties, it will probably be impossible, at least in the near term, to pursue this methodology in any rigorous way. Nevertheless, it does seem to offer a way of thinking about rationing decisions that could be useful in a less formal way, as, for instance, in the following scenario.

In a large HMO, the medical staff is asked to try to improve the allocation of expensive technologies. Each group of doctors responsible for a major medical technology (e.g., bone marrow transplant, hip replacement, and angioplasty) first characterizes the different patient subgroups that constitute the 10–15 percent of cases expected to benefit least. (Picking the lowest 15 percent of cases should be easy for experienced clinicians, although assigning a specific value for expected benefit is much harder.) They then make crude quantitative estimates of probabilities and benefits for these least promising patient groups in order to arrive at expected benefits per dollar. Representatives of each high-technology service then gather to examine and compare the expected benefits per dollar across technologies to see whether there are obviously higher payoffs in some than in others. Consistent with the overall budget constraint, a lowest acceptable value for expected benefits per dollar is identified and serves as the cutoff point, below which no further funding is provided for any technology. This ensures that the last (i.e., the least promising) case accepted for each intervention yields approximately the same benefit per dollar.

This admittedly rough-and-ready process would be assessed to see if it yielded more rational and equitable results than the traditional unstructured process that is typically based on a combination of politics, personalities, and chance. The procedure, even if it fails to solve the allocation problems, introduces a logical framework that at the very least should encourage physicians to think more systematically about resource allocation and perhaps stimulate others to improve on the basic approach that I am suggesting.

EFFECTS OF RATIONING ON PHYSICIANS AND PATIENTS

The imposition of an explicit rationing methodology will place physicians in a new and painful role. Instead of functioning solely as advocates for their patients, they will be required to make decisions involving tradeoffs between patients. The decision about how to treat an extremely premature infant, for example, will no longer be framed solely in terms of what is best for the patient and family, but rather in terms of the most effective use of limited resources. Squaring this new mandate with the physician's traditional ethical imperatives will be a challenge for the medical profession in the years ahead.

On the patient side, political pressures will surely develop as certain patients discover they are being denied forms of care that are being made available to others. Legislators and managed care administrators, who have a long history of abdicating responsibility when it comes to supporting specific allocation decisions, will be extremely sensitive to these forces.

Even under the best of circumstances, this approach to rationing cannot yield perfect decisions for all concerned. But it is only by testing such approaches in the real world that better ones may be developed. If rationing becomes the norm, there will inevitably be conflict between those who feel that decisions on care should be made explicit and obvious to patients and those who feel that implicit rationing is a kinder approach that spares the patient unnecessary psychological distress. The latter group will argue that the British system of "rationing by rationalization" is the more humane approach. Americans, however, are not likely to accept being kept in the dark on such important issues as their own health and the health of their families.

8

Cost Containment and the Cou

Establishing reasonable standards of care in the fiscally constrained environment that now confronts us will be a terribly difficult and contentious undertaking. Patients, health professionals, insurers, accrediting and licensing organizations, politicians, and government bureaucrats can all be expected to exert what pressure they can to see that standards of care meet their own expectations. There will be many battlegrounds in this war, but it is the courts that will ultimately decide how much freedom, if any, health care providers should have in offering a level of care that falls below standards considered desirable by experts. Two obvious areas in which plaintiffs will petition the courts are allegations of professional malpractice and of misrepresentation on the part of insurers regarding covered benefits. If the courts decide to weigh in heavily on the side of patients in either of these areas, the effort to restrain health care expenditures may be in serious trouble. In the long run, however, even the courts will have to acknowledge the altered fiscal realities of a new era.

To date, relatively few cases have come to trial in response to cost containment efforts, and almost all relate to the insurers' unwillingness to pay for "experimental" procedures or procedures that are not deemed "medically necessary." The majority of these cases have involved expensive procedures such as bone marrow or organ transplants for high-risk populations. These cases have been especially difficult to resolve because of the lack of standard criteria for determining what is experimental or medically necessary. The courts usually rely on the testimony of physicians, backed up by the evidence of current textbooks and journal articles, in assessing the validity of these determinations.[1] Variations in professional opinion and inconsistencies in the scientific literature may explain why the courts have reached contradictory conclusions about the same procedures. While 17 courts between 1990 and 1992 have ruled that autologous bone marrow transplant (ABMT) is not experimental, 12 courts in similar cases have denied coverage for ABMT, citing its experimental nature.[2]

A second, closely related issue confronts the courts in these cases. Did the beneficiary fully understand the terms of the contract and the likelihood that a particular therapy would be excluded from coverage? Although health insurance policies typically require that services be "medically necessary" to be covered and explicitly exclude "experimental" treatments, the courts often find that the insured could not reasonably be expected to understand the implications of these terms.[3] Among insurers, those with the most explicit definitions of coverage have the best chance of prevailing in court, but, overall, beneficiaries continue to win most cases.[4]

The nature of coverage disputes over experimental or unnecessary care is changing as insurers, particularly HMOs, increasingly require preapproval of procedures, thereby avoiding disputes after the fact about who is going to pay for them. As a result, the courts are called upon to intervene in life-or-death situations, where previously they only had to determine who was responsible for reimbursement after the service had been provided. In cases related to experimental treatment for terminally ill patients, the courts may be given the unenviable task of deciding whether a patient should be given a last chance to live.

A 1986 case, *Wickline v State of California*, first brought this problem into sharp focus. A woman's leg had to be amputated as a result of an alleged premature discharge after vascular surgery; her physician had requested an extended hospital stay, but the extension was denied by the insurer's utilization review program. The California Court of Appeals explicitly warned in its opinion that "A mistaken conclusion about medical necessity following retrospective review will result in the wrongful withholding of payment. An erroneous decision in a prospective review process, on the other hand, in practical consequences, results in the withholding of necessary care, potentially leading to a patient's permanent disability or death."[5]

A 1996 California law gives patients a stronger voice in obtaining approval for experimental or controversial care. A terminally ill patient denied care can now appeal to a panel of three outside physicians whose decisions are binding. The coauthor of the bill says that "the legislation will guarantee that decisions on treatment will be based on medical science, not on corporate profits." Delegating decisions to an impartial panel has obvious benefits, but it is hard to see how it solves the fundamental problem: defining "experimental" and "medically necessary."

As new medical technologies mature, typically over several years or more, experts generally develop consensus views about appropriate indications for their use. Such has been the case with heart and liver transplants, for example, which languished for many years in a morass of legal wrangling. The National Institutes of Health eventually convened a consensus panel, and its judgments have set the standard for the country as a whole. However, with a constant influx of new technologies, disputes over issues of safety, efficacy, and suitable patient candidates are likely to continue indefinitely. As the issues surrounding one intervention, such as bone marrow transplantation, are resolved, new issues over gene insertion, laboratory-grown tissue replacement, and hundreds of other emerging therapies can be anticipated.

MALPRACTICE AND MEDICAL NECESSITY

As difficult as it may be to establish the line dividing experimental care from non-experimental care, it is more difficult still to establish the line separating the medically necessary from the unnecessary, especially since the "standard of care" on which the courts must rely to assess medical necessity may not reflect the recent lowering of standards in response to rising cost concerns.[6] It is typically based on past medical practice, which means that the standard may carry with it costs in excess of current resource limitations.

In coverage disputes of the type I have discussed, the courts have been sympathetic to those who have been denied care. Their decisions indicate that the courts focus on the needs of the individual in the courtroom and do not give as much weight to the broad goals of society, such as the need to control health care costs.[7] In fact, the courts have yet to accept cost as a legitimate basis for denying care. Even in coverage decisions where the courts rule in favor of an insurer's decision to deny coverage, they do not necessarily condone the use of cost-effectiveness criteria. For example: in a recent case, *Barnett v Kaiser Foundation*, the court upheld a decision by Kaiser to deny coverage of a liver transplant for Ralph Barnett; Barnett had hepatitis B and had also been classified as "e-antigen positive," a condition that increased the risk that a new liver would become infected. One of the reasons the court gave for its finding in favor of Kaiser was that "there was no evidence the decision [by Kaiser's Advisory Board] was motivated by financial concerns for cost savings to the Kaiser Health Plan."[8] This cost-blind perspective brings the courts into direct conflict with cost containment efforts that necessitate new and lower standards of care.

UNDERSTANDING THE ROLE OF THE MALPRACTICE SYSTEM

Long before the added pressures of cost control, the malpractice system was a favorite target of health care reformers, attacked on the grounds that some patients receive unreasonably high awards, while other patients who have suffered equally receive nothing. These criticisms, however, assume that the goal of the malpractice system is to compensate injured patients and mete out equal justice to all, whereas it really has a much more limited goal: to discourage medically negligent behavior.

The argument against compensation as the rationale for negligence law goes back to the 1890s, when Justice Oliver Wendell Holmes pointed out that individuals could protect themselves more effectively against the costs of medical injuries simply by purchasing health insurance. It has been pointed out that the costs of the malpractice tort system are so high that only about 35 percent of the award reaches the injured party. Health insurance, by contrast, disburses 80 percent of the premium to patients with health insurance.[9] Malpractice law seems far more understandable when viewed as a means of warning physicians that negligence has economic consequences.

The legal meaning of negligence, however, is hard to pin down. Consider the classic definitions: "conduct which causes an unreasonably great risk of causing damage," or "conduct which falls below the standard established by law for the protection of others against unreasonably great risk of harm."[10] These definitions simply substitute other equally ambiguous terms for the word negligence. A more useful definition of negligence was formulated by Judge Learned Hand, who stated that "negligence occurs whenever it would cost less to prevent a mishap than to pay for the damages predicted to result from it."[11]

The practical applicability of this formulation can be demonstrated by an example.

A customer walking down the aisle of a supermarket knocks a jar of baby food to the floor, where it shatters. A few seconds later, another customer turns into the aisle, fails to see the puddle on the floor, slips and breaks a leg. It would not have been "reasonable" to expect that the owner of the market would station personnel in each aisle to offer continuous warnings about wet spots and to provide for instant cleanup. In this case, the cost of preventing the injury would far exceed the expected loss. Common sense would almost certainly lead a jury to conclude that negligence had not occurred. But if the wet spot had been left for 30 or 40 minutes, the verdict would be likely to go the other way, because the cost of policing the aisles at a longer interval is relatively low, and the likelihood of injury during that interval is considerably greater. As the cost of preventing a mishap rises and the likelihood becomes more remote, failing to avoid it becomes increasingly reasonable.[12]

As the supermarket case illustrates, someone who is injured is not automatically entitled to compensation even though everything about the injury itself is identical to that of another person who is compensated. What matters is that someone was negligent.

Medical negligence can be similarly equated with underinvesting in prevention of mishaps. When the amount of medical resources (time, materials, and professional skill) are provided at the level recommended by experts, there is virtually no risk of the physician being found guilty of negligence. Even high-risk patients treated in a standard manner have no basis for complaint if the outcome is bad, as long as reasonable resources have been devoted to avoiding the possibility of unfavorable outcomes.

While many physicians complain that there are too many malpractice claims, there is general agreement that many more incidents of malpractice occur than result in lawsuits being brought. Studies have shown that only 10 to 20 percent of negligent injuries lead to legal action.[13] Many are not brought for reasons that have no relationship to the validity of the claim, often because the patients don't know that the unfavorable outcome could have been avoided or don't want to jeopardize their relationship with their doctor. Further, a large number of malpractice claims are turned down by lawyers because they estimate that the award won't be large enough to justify their investment in the case. Nearly all cases of presumed negligence are taken on a contingency basis, with typically one-third of the award going to the lawyers.

To achieve complete deterrence, every instance of negligence should lead to a claim and every valid claim should lead to an appropriate award. Only then are providers fully motivated to improve their performance. But this ideal state does not exist. In fact, the current system provides only a modest encouragement to improve quality of care.

Critics point out that only a small percentage of culpable physicians are penalized in malpractice cases and that they are often insulated from the financial penalties through their malpractice insurance. Even physicians who have been found negligent on several occasions may be able to avoid losing insurance or facing increased premiums. The absence of so-called "experience rating" for malpractice insurance rates usually insulates the negligent physician from the consequences of malpractice, the fiscal burden being distributed across the entire pool of insured physicians.

MANAGED CARE GROUPS AND MALPRACTICE LITIGATION

Because relatively few cases of negligence result in claims, the door is opened for a managed care organization to maximize profits by anticipating and budgeting for malpractice suits on behalf of its employed physicians rather than investing in more and better staff or equipment. Consider the following example, related by a senior physician of a large managed care group. This dermatologist asked the hospital administration to make available certain expensive equipment and recently approved drugs that he felt were essential for the proper care of a group of patients with serious dermatologic problems. To make the investment decision, a group of administrators and lawyers met with the doctor and asked him what injury the patients would be likely to suffer without the added investment and what fraction of patients would suffer from being deprived of state-of-the art technology. The lawyers then estimated the number of claims that actually would be brought (probably about 10 percent of the patients who suffered) and the dollar payout that could be anticipated for each injury. When the total anticipated payout for claims was found to be substantially below the costs of new equipment and better drugs, the managed care group decided to forgo the improved care and instead pay the claims that might be brought. Similar decisions will be made in other managed care organizations if they choose to put profits ahead of patient welfare.

The deterrent effect of malpractice awards has been further attenuated for HMOs by the Employment Retirement Insurance Security Act (ERISA) of 1974, which makes it difficult for patients to bring suit against employer-sponsored and self-funded managed care plans. This unusual protection from suit is based in a broad preemption of state insurance laws dealing with malpractice and employee benefits.[14] The protection extends to liability claims even if the claim is based on "bad faith" or "breach of contract."

However, a 1995 decision by the Supreme Court is likely to modify this blanket protection.[15] The Court ruled that self-funded plans and contracting agents of employer plans have no absolute guarantee of preemption from state laws.[16] Also, in 1997 legislation was introduced in Congress, with 170 cosponsors, that would weaken the ERISA protections and give many employees the right to sue both their managed care providers and the employers who contract with them.[17] Indeed, it is quite clear that the framers of the ERISA legislation intended primarily to protect union pension funds and group legal service plans and never envisioned that ERISA would be used as a means to insulate managed health care plans against malpractice claims.

TRENDS FOR THE FUTURE

As standards of care evolve in response to budget constraints, conflicts between the old and new criteria will inevitably arise. In the near future, for instance, the number of bad outcomes in the course of hospital stays can be expected to increase as a result of briefer hospital stays, fewer intensive care beds, reduced availability of medical specialists, less expert nursing care, and other features of a cost-constrained health care system. In this environment, long-established guidelines based on expert opinion will no longer provide dependable guidance for physicians and other health care professionals trying to render cost-effective care and still remain on the safe side of the malpractice threshold. Patients will be equally at a loss to judge whether an unsuccessfully treated illness is due to a lowering of systemwide standards or to the individual professional's negligence. Defining acceptable levels of medical care will be the bane of judges and juries for years to come.

Part Three

Molecular Medicine

Comes into Its Own

2020 and Beyond

The wellspring of many of the therapeutic advances that will dominate medicine in the second quarter of the next century will be the science of molecular biology. Although this discipline will already have yielded important diagnostic tools by the early part of the century, the arrival on the scene of molecular therapies like gene insertion will raise medical care to an entirely new level. Indeed, the tools of molecular biology appear to have such potential to unlock the mysteries of disease that the age-old dream of a disease-free world no longer seems outlandish. It is obviously much too soon to predict with any accuracy what can be expected from molecular medicine, but I attempt to provide here a glimpse of some of the more intriguing possibilities. A critical policy question that remains unanswered is what effect this advancing technology will have on costs; indications are that, at least until they are fully mature, molecular therapies will be expensive. The first generation of therapies could aggravate cost problems by turning some diseases that are now rapidly lethal into chronic ones, thereby putting new demands on over-stretched health care budgets.

Assuming that these troubled waters can be navigated successfully, there is at least a chance that there are calmer seas ahead. By the year 2050, the conquest of many diseases could be a reality and health-care costs brought under control. The resulting increase in longevity, perhaps forty years or more, could bring into play an entirely new set of problems caused by generations of healthy humans who refuse to die.

9

Molecular Medicine:

A New Era of Therapy

Many of the early successes of molecular medicine, as I discussed in chapter 4, have been in the diagnostic arena, particularly in the ability to screen patients for genetic predisposition to disease. As the achievements of molecular medicine begin to accumulate in the next century, physicians will be able to move beyond simply warning patients about their chances of developing diseases. They will have the tools to alter the underlying genetic causes and thereby offer relief from even such relentless killers as heart disease, stroke, and cancer.

The discussions in this chapter provide highly selective and cursory sketches of some of the most promising early research fronts in molecular medicine. The "hot" areas of research will undoubtedly shift many times even before the end of the next decade, and the examples presented here should be taken simply as evidence of molecular biology's unprecedented potential for therapeutic success. Many of the therapeutic techniques discussed have not yet moved beyond the laboratory bench, and some may not prove to be clinically practical, but it seems reasonable to assume that many will reach the bedside within the next few decades.

Whenever a gene's link to a particular disease process can be established, it becomes possible, at least theoretically, to devise specific therapeutic interventions. By 1997, genes and the proteins they encode had been identified for a wide range of diseases, including amyotrophic lateral sclerosis (Lou Gehrig's disease), Huntington's disease, cystic fibrosis, epilepsy, and glaucoma. Potential therapies to correct these and other disorders can be targeted at several different stages of the progression from abnormal gene to abnormal protein, that is, by:

· inserting normal genes to compensate for missing or damaged genes
· regulating the mechanisms by which genes are activated and shut off
· interfering with the process of gene expression, especially targeting the role of messenger RNA
· mitigating or neutralizing the effects of missing or abnormal proteins

GENE THERAPY

Perhaps the most dramatic and ambitious of these strategies is gene therapy. This approach typically involves delivery to cells of normal genes that encode for normal proteins. To insert a normal gene into cells to compensate for a missing or defective one, the gene is usually transferred into a vector, typically a virus that has been modified so that it can't replicate, which in turn invades specific cells during cell division and delivers its cargo of genetic material. The goal is for the new gene to take the place of the disordered gene in directing the production of a protein required for normal physiologic function.

In 1995, an advisory committee to the National Institutes of Health determined that gene therapy had been oversold. The public, it concluded, has been encouraged into unwarranted enthusiasm about the prospects of successful gene replacement when, in fact, clinical efficacy has not been definitively demonstrated in any gene therapy. The co-chair of the committee commented that "basic science was being neglected as enthusiasts race to join the gene therapy club." More attention, the panel advised, should be paid to fundamental questions such as improving the efficiency of the vectors that carry genes into the cell and to gene regulation.[1]

A host of problems remains to be solved, including inserting the genes into the right cells, achieving an adequate and sustained level of gene expression (i.e., production of the desired protein), and replacing the genes when the host cells die. Many members of the scientific community remain optimistic, however, that these problems will eventually be overcome and the door opened to effective therapy. A clinical study reported in November 1997 gives hope that progress may be faster than has generally been thought. That study demonstrated that gene therapy can stimulate the growth of collateral vessels around severely obstructed arteries in the leg and result in a dramatic and lasting clinical improvement. Commenting on this work, Stuart Orkin, a leading expert on gene therapy research, noted, "It is one of the first, if not the first, times that gene therapy has resulted in a clinical improvement." The recent report of successful synthesis of artificial chromosomes may provide a way to circumvent some of the problems of gene insertion by providing a stable, natural vehicle with which to deliver therapeutic genes to cells.[2]

BLOCKING GENE EXPRESSION

Another promising strategy consists of interfering with the mechanisms by which either a normal or a faulty gene communicates its instructions. So-called "antisense" agents do just this and in so doing block the synthesis of the protein that has been specified by the gene. Antisense compounds can either bind to the gene itself or to the messenger RNA (mRNA) that carries the encoded information, leading to its destruction. Another way of destroying the mRNA is by the use of "ribozymes," RNA molecules that can bind to and cut messenger RNA into pieces. Research on this front is being pursued in many laboratories and for many diseases: cancer, hypertension, coronary artery disease, AIDS, and leukemia. Although there has been concern that antisense agents might not be effective when delivered systemically, researchers have announced initial success in intravenous delivery of an antisense drug to treat Crohn's disease, a chronic inflammatory disease of the lower intestinal tract.[3]

DEALING WITH THE PROTEIN PRODUCTS OF GENES

Yet another approach to therapy lies in the administration of agents that compensate for the proteins that a scrambled or missing gene cannot produce. A defective gene can result in disease either because no protein at all is expressed or because the protein that is expressed is altered in such a way that it is non-functional. Specific drugs could therefore be designed to either supply a missing protein or reduce the toxicity of a damaged protein.

ALTERING THE WAY CELLS COMMUNICATE WITH EACH OTHER

Molecular therapies can be aimed at the signaling processes both within and between cells. Cells do not function in isolation: they must communicate with other cells to carry out complex physiological processes. This signaling can take place either between neighboring cells that make up an organ or by means of hormones such as insulin and estrogen, which travel through the bloodstream to a matching receptor at a remote site. When activated, cell receptors set into motion a process that carries the message through the cell membrane and into the cell, where they can, for example,

trigger growth or initiate metabolic activity. All messenger molecules represent opportunities for therapeutic interventions.

TAKING AIM AT THE GENES RESPONSIBLE FOR CANCER

Normal cell growth is controlled by a battery of genes whose products either induce or suppress cell division. Proto-oncogenes are a
family of different proteins that perform essential functions such
as gene regulation, regulation of cell reproduction, and growth.
Cancer can be caused when one or more of these genes are converted into cancer-causing oncogenes, resulting in persistent stimulation and uncontrolled cell growth. New therapeutic approaches
will rely on controlling the flow of misinformation from oncogenes by many of the strategies discussed above.

Oncogenes, however, are only a part of the cancer story. Recent
research indicates that malignancies also develop because of abnormalities in genes whose specialized function it is to control
normal cell multiplication. When these genes, called "tumor
suppressor genes," mutate and lose their control function, uncontrolled replication follows. Loss or mutation of one tumor-
suppressor gene, designated the p53 gene, is thought to contribute
to the development of perhaps 50 percent of all cancers. The presence of an oncogene combined with the loss of a tumor-suppressor
gene gives tumor cells a tremendous growth advantage over
normal cells.

In addition to targeting the direct role of genes in the development and control of cancer, researchers are investigating a wide
array of strategies that exploit the discoveries of molecular biology
in arresting cancerous cell growth. A critical pathway for signal
transmission through the cell membrane and into the cell itself has
recently been discovered, and it has been shown that a class of
proteins required for this pathway is abnormal in certain cancers,

including leukemia. An abnormality in these "G-proteins" appears to play a critical role in the uncontrolled cell growth characteristic of malignant tumors, and it is possible that drugs could be designed to compensate for the abnormal proteins.

Excellent experimental progress is also being made in dealing with metastases—tumors that have spread to other organs from their original sites and often indicate a poor prognosis. One intriguing approach limits the growth of such metastases by curtailing their blood supply. Rapidly growing malignant tissues require an ever-larger supply of nutrients and oxygen, which is provided by a steady growth of new blood vessels. Inhibitory compounds produced by genetic engineering, known as anti-angiogenic factors, suppress the growth of new blood vessels and may prove effective in keeping the metastases of some tumors in check even when they cannot be completely cured. Colon and breast cancer appear to be particularly promising targets for this therapy. The discovery of a gene that directly suppresses the development of metastases has opened still another window on therapy, and a combination of gene therapy and administration of anti-angiogenic agents may prove more valuable than either one alone.

The body's natural immune defenses can be put to work to fight tumors in the same way that they fight off infections. Tumor cells, we are learning, carry pathologic proteins on their surface, but these proteins can escape recognition by the body's immunologic defense system. When they are isolated from a tumor, however, large quantities of antibodies specific to these proteins can be produced in the laboratory. The antibodies can then be coupled with a payload of chemotherapy agents. When this chemotherapy complex is administered, the antibody zeroes in on the cells for which it has an affinity and releases its load of cell-destructive toxin. This technique has the advantage of attacking only the tumor cells without harming normal cells. Successes to date have been modest, but the concept appears sound. Cancer cells may also yield to another immunologic approach: vaccines made from the individual's own cancer cells, combined with substances that stimulate the body's immune system, are under study in the hope that the cancer cells can be destroyed by the body's own lymphocytes without the use of additional toxic agents.

One of the great mysteries of cancer has been the fact that cancer cells can continue to divide and replicate themselves almost indefinitely into new generations, whereas normal cells lose this ability after about fifty generations. An enzyme called telomerase, which appears to be essential to the "immortality" of cancer cells, thus provides another valuable biochemical target. Each of a normal cell's chromosomes has a cap at each end made up of structures called telomeres. These caps protect the genes in the chromosome from injury and allow cell division to proceed normally. As cells divide, the telomere cap shortens at each replication; when the cap shortens beyond a certain threshold, multiplication of the cell is arrested. Cancerous cells are different. They contain telomerase, which rebuilds the telomere cap and maintains the ability of the cell to divide indefinitely. Because telomerase is present in most cancer cells and suppressed in most normal cells, it provides an inviting target for drug therapy. Agents that interfere with telomerase activity but exert minimal effect on normal tissues are under investigation.

Because most tumors are solid masses, their structure limits the penetration of therapeutic agents, even the targeted agents discussed above, into the tumor tissue. How to reach all of the cancer cells is a critical problem because even a single surviving cell can perpetuate the cancer. And even if an agent can reach the surface of each cell in the tumor mass, it may be unable to penetrate into the cell, to attack cellular proteins, or into the nucleus and its DNA. A particularly challenging problem will be finding a technique for permeating the tumor mass completely. Biotechnology firms are hard at work on this and related problems in hopes of reaping the rewards that can be anticipated from a new generation of safe and effective cancer therapies.

THE ROLE OF GENETICALLY
EXPRESSED PROTEINS IN OTHER DISEASES

Our growing understanding of genetic abnormalities and the way they produce disease through missing or defective proteins extends well beyond cancer into a broad spectrum of human disease. What follows are snapshots of some major diseases in which the responsible gene has been located and the normal protein it expresses in healthy individuals has been identified. The usual cause of disease is the production of a mutant version of the normal protein, which cannot perform its normal functions. The rate of gene discovery and characterization appears to be accelerating, and the next few years will see many additions to this list.

Amyotrophic Lateral Sclerosis Amyotrophic lateral sclerosis (ALS), known as Lou Gehrig's disease, is a progressive disease of the motor neurons in the brain and spinal cord that causes increasing difficulty in swallowing, speaking, and all other motor functions. Recently, the mutant gene responsible for the disease in familial cases has been identified. The normal gene encodes for a detoxification enzyme that safely eliminates free radicals formed during metabolism. (Free radicals are chemically unstable molecules that react with and damage proteins, DNA, and membranes, causing cellular injury.) The mutated version of the enzyme is not as efficient in detoxifying these radicals, and this deficiency apparently accounts for the nerve damage characteristic of ALS.[4]

Huntington's Disease Huntington's disease gives rise to a range of disabling symptoms, including involuntary, spasmodic body movement and severe mental disturbance. It is a fatal disease that is characterized by severe damage to certain specialized parts of the brain, with widespread damage or destruction of nerves. The gene responsible for Huntington's was discovered in 1993, but scientists were initially unable to determine the protein abnormality it caused. In 1997 it was discovered that the defective gene in Huntington's contains a "stutter" in its DNA encoding that puts extra copies of the amino acid glutamine into the protein it expresses. These glutamine-heavy molecules clump together and eventually reach a trigger point at which they begin migrating from the cytoplasm into the nucleus of brain cells, resulting in cell death. Researchers have already begun searching for the drugs that might prevent the defective protein molecules from joining together.[5]

Epilepsy   The gene whose defect is responsible for a rare form of progressive myoclonus epilepsy has recently been identified and, on its heels, the protein that the normal gene codes for, cystatin B. This protein, a protease inhibitor, exerts a protective action by blocking the action of protein-cleaving enzymes that otherwise might cause damage to cells. When a genetic abnormality leads to a deficiency of cystatin B, epilepsy occurs. Discovery of the role of protease inhibition in this rare form of epilepsy raises the possibility that uncontrolled activity of protein-cleaving enzymes may contribute to other, more common epilepsies. A wide range of protease inhibitors are now under study as potential therapeutic agents.

Cystic Fibrosis   Cystic fibrosis is one of the most common inherited diseases in the United States. Although the disease compromises many organs, lung infections and respiratory failure are nearly always the cause of death. Improved antibiotics have led to longer life but do not strike at the cause of the disease. The primary abnormality in cystic fibrosis is a defect in the ability to move chloride across certain cell membranes, such as those in the lung and sweat glands. In lung tissue, the normal movement of chloride from the blood to the airway serves to pull water into the lung spaces, thus keeping the mucus in the bronchial tubes thin enough to trap bacteria and other particles and to be coughed up through the throat. The importance of the defect in chloride movement was revealed by the discovery of a gene and its expressed protein, called cystic fibrosis transmembrane regulator, which maintains a channel for chloride and water migration through the cell membrane. The mutant gene and its abnormal protein eliminate this channeling capability and cause the mucus in the lung to become thick and difficult to expel.[6] Although this finding appeared to account sufficiently for the serious, recurrent infections in cystic fibrosis, the story is more complex. The high chloride concentration in the mucus has also been shown to block the effects of a natural antibiotic that lines the lungs of normal individuals, thus contributing to the high rate of infections in cystic fibrosis patients.[7]

Glaucoma   Glaucoma, a condition in which the pressure in the fluid of the eye becomes elevated, damages the optic nerve and causes loss of vision and even blindness. Because glaucoma often develops without symptoms, many patients suffer irreversible vision loss before a diagnosis can be made and appropriate drug therapy instituted. A genetic abnormality and resulting expression of a protein (TIGR) now appears to be responsible for juvenile glaucoma. Based on this discovery, a screening test should soon be available that will identify patients at risk. Although juvenile glaucoma accounts for only about 1 percent of all glaucoma cases, it appears that the screening test could identify at least 3 percent of potential glaucoma cases. This could mean early diagnosis and therapeutic intervention with pressure-lowering drugs for as many as one hundred thousand people in the United States.[8]

MOLECULAR APPROACHES TO
CARDIOVASCULAR DISEASE AND STROKE

Coronary Artery Disease Coronary artery disease, characterized by narrowing of the coronary arteries supplying the heart, remains one of the most troublesome medical complaints, despite continuing advances in prevention and treatment. The classic symptom is a constricting chest pain called angina pectoris, which often radiates down the left arm and sometimes into the neck and jaw. The pain, which is usually precipitated by exercise or stress, results from reduced blood flow to a portion of the heart; it is often severe enough to prevent sufferers from performing normal activities. Preventive efforts includes such familiar measures as regular exercise, eliminating smoking, observing a diet low in fat and cholesterol, and, if necessary, drug therapy to lower high blood cholesterol levels. Unfortunately, current measures are often ineffective, and attention has turned to molecular approaches targeted at the causes of coronary artery disease.

One approach is designed to alter the way the body stores and metabolizes cholesterol. This strategy has so far focused on a small number of patients with a genetic abnormality that causes extremely high levels of cholesterol in the blood. These patients lack the capacity to clear the low-density lipoprotein (LDL) form of cholesterol from the blood, because they have too few LDL receptors on cells (particularly liver cells) that perform this task. They can have cholesterol levels as high as 1,000 mg/dL (normal is less than 200 mg/dL) and are prone to narrowing of the coronary arteries and heart attacks as early as the teen years.

In one experimental approach to this problem, a normal LDL gene was introduced into liver cells using gene therapy to increase the number of LDL receptors present in the liver. When the treated liver cells were infused back into the patient, a decrease in serum

LDL was observed.[9] If this therapy eventually proves effective in patients with grossly elevated LDL levels, it will also open the door to treatment of patients with less severe elevations of cholesterol.

Currently, the treatment for seriously clogged arteries is either a coronary artery bypass graft or angioplasty, a procedure in which a catheter with a small balloon at its tip is inserted into the affected vessel and advanced to the point of obstruction. The balloon is then expanded to crack open the hardened vessel wall and to dilate the opening. Because the coronary arteries are traumatized during angioplasty, they release reparative growth factors that cause arterial smooth muscle cells to proliferate, thus narrowing the blood vessel and reducing blood supply again. Research is now focusing on methods to break the link between injury and cellular overgrowth in the artery. Efforts are being made to design antisense drugs that will inactivate the growth-factor gene and thus block the synthesis of the factors themselves. Genes that encode proteins which protect against proliferation are also being inserted directly into coronary vessel cells in laboratory animals.

Repairing Damaged Heart Muscle   Heart attacks strike when a narrowed coronary artery becomes completely obstructed by a blood clot. A scrambling of the heart's electrical control mechanisms can produce sudden death by arresting the pumping action of the heart. Even if the patient survives, a section of the heart muscle dies, and the pumping action of the heart can be impaired to the point of causing congestive heart failure. As the reduction in pumping capacity progresses, the excretion of salt and water by the kidney is impaired, and pulmonary edema and swelling of the lower legs result. The standard treatment of congestive heart failure has been administration of digitalis to improve the pumping efficiency of the heart and diuretics to promote salt and water excretion. These measures work well for many patients but not for all.

Efforts are now being directed toward replacing the damaged

muscle. In one approach, skeletal muscle cells or fetal heart cells are transferred into the damaged portion of the heart with the aims of generating growth and reviving the function of the flagging heart muscle.[10] In another, connective tissue cells that form the scaffold of the heart but do not normally contribute to pumping are being explored as a potential source of heart muscle replacement.[11] The challenge will be to genetically alter the structural cells so that they can function as muscle cells and restore normal pumping function.

Stimulating New Vessel Growth in Vascular Disease   Patients with a blockage in the femoral artery of the leg experience intense pain during walking because of inadequate oxygenation of the leg muscles. Progressive reduction in blood flow can eventually require amputation of the leg. To prevent this outcome, three surgical approaches are possible. The obstructing fatty deposits can be removed; an angioplasty may be undertaken; or the area of obstruction may be bypassed with a graft. These approaches are often only partially effective and have created an obvious need for a new generation of therapies.

The most promising new approach builds upon the observation that when arteries are blocked by disease, the body tries to compensate for the reduced blood flow by forming new vessels to carry blood around the blocked or partially blocked area. Typically, however, these so-called collateral vessels are too few and too small to compensate for the deficiency in flow or to prevent damage to the surrounding tissue. Several years ago it was discovered that a naturally occurring substance, called vascular endothelial growth factor (VEGF), is responsible for promoting growth of collateral vessels. This finding led to the idea that the gene for this growth-enhancing protein could be introduced into the muscle cells in the wall of the obstructed vessel and there induce new growth sufficient to allow adequate blood flow around the obstruction.[12] The strategy faces many of the same obstacles as other attempts at gene insertion, except that in muscle tissue no vector is required to deliver the genetic material, which can enter cells as "naked" DNA.[13]

In a small but potentially pivotal study, genetic treatment of severe arterial disease in the lower extremities has been shown to induce a marked proliferation of collateral vessels and an increase in blood flow sufficient to relieve severe pain and in some cases to avoid the need for amputation. The treatment halted both gangrene and ulcers in all but one of the ten patients treated.[14] Success with leg vessels will almost certainly be followed by attempts to treat partially occluded coronary vessels—in effect, a nonsurgical coronary bypass. Such a procedure could reduce the widespread use of angioplasty and bypass surgery for heart disease. Only more extensive studies will tell whether the enthusiastic initial appraisals can be supported.

Stroke   Strokes are common and devastating brain injuries, brought on most often by a clot suddenly occluding an artery that supplies a part of the brain with its essential oxygen flow. Common clinical findings are weakness or paralysis of one side of the body, loss of memory, and compromised vision and speech. The death rate is 10 to 15 percent, and another 20 percent of patients require lengthy hospitalization. Until recently there was almost nothing that could be done to limit or repair the brain damage caused by strokes. Imagine, then, the impact of evolving research that might one day make these "brain attacks" as susceptible to effective intervention as heart attacks.

The mainstay of current therapy is the administration of a bioengineered drug, tissue plasminogen activator (tPA), to dissolve the clot and restore blood flow.[15] To be effective the therapy must be instituted within a brief window of time after the stroke. When this is possible, about half of the patients are spared any permanent disability, but tPA does induce complications in some patients and is not an ideal form of therapy.[16]

The next wave of therapeutic agents is developing from the finding that cellular responses to the initial injury set off a chain reaction of catastrophic events that affects a substantially larger area of the brain. Cutting off the blood supply to an area of brain cells by occlusion of a vessel leads to cell death within minutes in the region totally deprived of oxygen, but surrounding tissues whose blood supply is partially compromised also suffer damage. The diminished blood supply sets into motion a cascade of destructive events, starting with damage to the cell membranes, which leads to an outpouring of glutamate. Too much glutamate, in turn, causes calcium ions to flood into cells where it activates enzymes that cause cells to self-destruct. Drugs that interfere with this sequence of events, so-called neuroprotective drugs, are under development by many companies. They include antioxidants to neutralize toxic "free radical" molecules, calcium channel blockers to prevent excess influx of calcium into cells, and agents that block the toxic effects of excess glutamate.[17]

Current thinking envisions that future stroke therapy will consist of tPA (or a similar agent) combined with neuroprotective drugs, but their success will continue to rely on the speed with which stroke victims can be treated. Improved MRI technology will help by allowing physicians to pinpoint the oxygen-deprived portions of the brain in a matter of minutes. A tougher problem will be getting the word out to the public at large that every second counts in recognizing stroke and transporting stroke victims to the emergency room.

ADVANCES IN IMMUNOLOGY AND INFECTIOUS DISEASE

Autoimmune diseases   In healthy individuals, the immune system reacts only to foreign proteins such as bacteria or viruses, which it destroys to protect the organism. The major weapons in this immunologic defense are white blood cells of a type called lymphocytes. The body produces billions of lymphocytes, each capable of recognizing a specific protein. Two major types of lymphocytes are the B-lymphocytes, which produce antibodies against foreign proteins, and T-lymphocytes, which send out chemical signals that activate a variety of defense mechanisms. As an individual's pool of lymphocytes grows in embryo, the body can identify and screen out those lymphocytes that have the dangerous potential to recognize and destroy its own tissues. This screening process allows the individual to become fully tolerant to "self" while retaining the ability to attack non-self proteins.

In autoimmune diseases, some lymphocytes mistakenly identify certain normal tissues as foreign and make them the target of attack—the resulting disease being determined by the type of tissues under attack. For example, when rogue lymphocytes destroy the insulin-secreting cells of the pancreas, the result is diabetes; when they destroy the proteins of joint surfaces, they cause rheumatoid arthritis. Other common autoimmune diseases include multiple sclerosis, lupus erythematosus, psoriasis, and certain types of hyperthyroidism and destructive vascular disease. Thus, a group of puzzling disorders that at one time seemed unrelated to one another are now known to share the same fundamental etiology. This finding has set into motion an intense search for the mechanisms that cause lymphocytes to misbehave.

One of the most suggestive findings comes from recent studies of juvenile diabetes in animals. These studies indicate that the normal immunologic attack on an invading bacterium can lead to a costly case of mistaken identity that culminates in juvenile diabetes. The story starts with the discovery of a link between juvenile diabetes (type 1 diabetes) and infection with the relatively benign Coxsackie virus, a common cause of colds and sore throats in children. After the Coxsackie virus is broken down into small chains of amino acids by the immune system, some of those chains themselves also come under attack. But the structure of the viral fragments under attack is so similar to the structure of a protein on the insulin-producing cells of the pancreas that these cells are also treated as foreign by the immune system—and are damaged or destroyed. Juvenile diabetes is thought to be the result of this "molecular mimicry," and the search is on to see whether additional reactions between an infectious agent and a protein component of other tissue, such as a joint surface, may be involved in triggering other autoimmune diseases.[18]

The current treatment of autoimmune disorders focuses on inhibiting the action of the disease-causing lymphocytes. Prednisone and other immunosuppressive drugs are the agents of choice, but they inhibit not only the offending lymphocytes but essential, normal ones as well. Because control of autoimmune disease is accomplished by weakening the body's immune defenses, susceptibility to infection is increased. Immunosuppressive steroids also have side effects, including the development of cataracts, diabetes, and osteoporosis, which limit their usefulness. More recently, however, the tools of molecular biology have been brought to bear on the problem of selectively attacking the rogue lymphocytes. For example, a specific set of lymphocytes has been identified as a cause of psoriasis. Treatment with antibodies that target these particular cells has been moderately successful.[19]

Another approach, called oral tolerization, makes use of the fact that the immune system of the gastrointestinal tract suppresses hostile attacks on foreign proteins ingested as part of the diet, even when the same proteins injected intravenously or into muscle cause a severe immune response.[20] If the gastrointestinal tract did not in some way block the body's normal reaction to foreign proteins, ingestion of food would set into motion a disastrous immune reaction. This phenomenon has led to experiments designed to induce "tolerization" for a protein that would otherwise produce a hostile immune response. Early experiments in patients with multiple sclerosis who were fed a protein from the surface of bovine nerve cells is reported to reduce the severity of the attacks typical of the disease.[21] Similarly favorable results have been reported after feeding collagen extracts to patients with rheumatoid arthritis.[22] Recent studies in experimental animals have suggested possible mechanisms that account for the oral tolerization process in multiple sclerosis, encephalitis, arthritis, and diabetes.[23]

Expanding Horizons of Organ Transplantation   When a patient's vital organs are diseased or damaged beyond repair, a transplant may offer the only hope of recovery. Yet the transplantation of human organs poses a daunting array of logistical and ethical obstacles, depending as it does on the availability of a donor with a suitable tissue match to the recipient and on the rapid transportation of the donated organ for surgery. Xenotransplantation, the transplantation of animal organs into humans, could circumvent many of these difficulties, but it has been stymied by the problem of immunologic rejection of the foreign tissue. However, insertion of human genes into animal organs may make them suitable for transplantation into humans without provoking significant immune reactions. As a result of the gene insertion, animal tissues can express human histocompatibility antigens that fool the immune system into regarding the tissue as human. Work in this area must be undertaken with caution, because unknown infectious agents might be present in the animal organs and prove difficult or impossible to eradicate when transferred to a human host. Transplantation of organs from a primate such as a baboon is probably far riskier than transplanting pig organs, since primates have closer biological similarities to man and are therefore more likely to harbor an infection that can cross species.

Antibiotic-Resistant Infections I have vivid memories of my episode of "double pneumonia" as a twelve-year-old in the 1930s, debilitated by a severe cough, malaise, loss of appetite, and a high fever. No drugs, not even the sulfa drugs, were available; mustard plasters were applied to my chest in the vague hope of "stirring up the circulation" in my lungs. The local doctor came to my home each day, examined me sympathetically, and left. Everyone seemed to be aware that soon either the fever would break and I would recover, or it would continue unabated and I would die. This recollection underlines the striking contrast between that pre-antibiotic era and the era of now-familiar "miracle" drugs like penicillin and streptomycin. The dreaded organisms such as pneumococci, streptococci and staphylococci, and the tubercle bacillus seemed, until recently, to be defeated by the arts of modern medicinal chemistry.

But a disturbing thing has happened. In recent years, resistant organisms have emerged in ever-increasing numbers, and we face the prospect of a return to an age of untreatable infections. The Darwinian process of natural selection has subverted efforts at control by favoring the proliferation of strains of bacteria resistant to antibiotics. Reliably effective agents are becoming scarce, partly because the pharmaceutical industry has depended on just a handful of drug groups, which have been repeatedly modified to deal with the problem of resistance. Some 16 basic compounds have been modified in about 160 ways, but the bacteria keep developing ways to circumvent their effects. No major new class of antibiotics has been discovered in the last two decades, and variants on the old ones are losing their punch. One dangerous organism, a strain of intestine-dwelling enterococcus, is no longer vulnerable to any antibiotic. What is worse, it has the potential ability to transfer its resistance trait to even more dangerous bacteria.[24]

The prospect of raging epidemics caused by resistant organisms has given impetus to new research efforts within many drug companies. The result has been experimental work on whole new classes of antibiotics.[25] Instead of screening thousands of compounds to see which might be effective against an organism, researchers are turning to molecular biology to scope out the vulnerable aspects of the organism's genome. Molecular biologists are, for example, working to identify the genes that determine a bacterium's degree of virulence and to identify proteins it produces which could be used in the development of vaccines. Such efforts should reveal a host of possible targets for drug intervention, including the proteins induced by the "virulent" genes. Efforts are also under way to undermine the mechanisms by which bacteria protect themselves under a coating of lipids on their surface.[26] Without those protective sheaths, bacteria may become easy targets for the body's natural defense mechanisms.

One notable recent success in the molecular war on infectious disease has been with *Helicobacter pylori*, introduced in chapter 1 as the bacterial cause of most peptic ulcers. New computer-based techniques for deciphering DNA sequences have permitted the complete sequencing of the *H. pylori* genome, providing scientists with a wealth of information about how the bacterium survives in the hostile environment of the human gastrointestinal tract and how its various defenses might be undermined. Some of the genes identified are responsible for the organism's ability to burrow into the stomach wall and adhere to cells there; others pump out the hydrochloric acid that enters the organism from the host's digestive fluids, and still others continually transform the composition of the organism's surface coating in order to elude recognition by the body's immune response.

As the defense mechanisms of this and other pathogenic bacteria are elucidated at the molecular level, new, highly specific drug therapies will become feasible. However, it may still be five or ten years before new drugs based on these insights become available. When they do, they can be expected to carry hefty price tags to compensate for the extensive research and clinical trials required to develop and test them. In the meantime, the treatment of bacterial diseases will go through a period in which effective therapy can no longer be taken for granted.

Viral Infections   Major advances are also anticipated for the treatment of viral diseases, both familiar ones like HIV infection and those which may emerge in the future. One important approach introduced recently in AIDS treatment, and which is potentially valuable in other diseases, blocks replication of the virus by means of drugs called protease inhibitors. These agents inhibit the formation of proteins required for the structural integrity of the virus. Also under development is a new class of drugs, known as nucleoside analogs, that inhibit the process by which viruses replicate their genetic material. A further therapeutic strategy will be to block the activity of the harmful proteins expressed by the virus.

New and successful treatment of viral diseases will involve a multi-pronged approach using these and other new therapies based on a growing understanding of the genetic code of the infectious viruses. The therapies will reduce viral burden (the absolute number of viruses in the infected patient) but cannot be expected to completely eliminate viral infection. Complete eradication of a virus and long-term cure of infection may depend on virus-specific therapies combined with enhancement of the patient's normal immune response. Ultimately, the goal will be to prevent viral infection from developing in the first place through new immunization techniques customized against emergent viruses as soon as they are recognized as causes of disease.

LIMITATIONS OF MOLECULAR THERAPIES AND EFFECTS ON COSTS

Molecular therapies for most diseases, at least initially, will be far less than optimal and may not provide speedy cures, with the result that costs of care will remain substantial. Some of the factors limiting the success of gene therapies and mitigating any desired cost savings are these:

- Gene therapy will be only partially effective because it is difficult to get the genetic material into enough cells—and the right cells—to have a therapeutic effect for a prolonged period. This limitation is especially significant for cancers, since even a single untreated cell can result in recurrence of the disease. Drugs targeted at regulation of gene expression encounter obstacles in entering the cell membrane and have even more trouble penetrating the cell nucleus where key targets for treatment lie.
- Molecular-based drug therapies may produce unexpected adverse reactions that will limit the drugs' usefulness and may create a need for additional care.
- Many patients for whom there was no previously successful treatment will now be candidates for new treatments, putting increased demands on health care resources.
- Even when treatment is effective, it may turn an acute illness, which runs a rapid course, into a chronic disease, extending the duration and expenses of therapy. Multi-drug therapy for AIDS is a striking example of this phenomenon. There is no doubt that new drugs are slowing progress of the illness, but experts believe that complete cure is still many years away.

In perhaps 25 to 30 years, many of these problems should be resolved, as a growing understanding of the genes and their protein products permits more precisely targeted therapies. With this development, medicine will be within sight of an era in which the prevention or prompt cure of disease achieves wide-ranging success.

10

On the Threshold of Utopia:
Approaching 2050

Exactly where we will stand in the war against disease by the year 2050 is of course impossible to say. But if developments in research maintain their current pace, it seems likely that a combination of improved attention to dietary and environmental factors along with advances in gene therapy and protein-targeted drugs will have virtually eliminated most major classes of disease.

From an economic standpoint, the best news may be that these accomplishments could be accompanied by a drop in costs. After a continuing rise in expenditures during the early years of the molecular medicine era, a plateau should be reached. Costs may even fall as diseases are brought under control using pinpointed, short-term therapies that are the fruits of the intellectual and social capital currently being expended on research. There will be many fewer hospitals, and surgical procedures will be largely restricted to the treatment of accidents and other forms of trauma. Spending on non-acute care, both in nursing facilities and in homes, will also fall sharply as the healthy elderly lead normal or near-normal lives until close to death.

One result of medicine's success in controlling disease will be a dramatic increase in life expectancy. How great that increase will be is a highly speculative matter, but it is worth noting that medical science has already helped to make the very old (currently defined as those over 85 years of age) the fastest-growing segment of the population. Between 1960 and 1995, the U.S. population as a whole increased by about 45 percent, whereas the segment over 85 years of age grew by almost 300 percent.[1] And there has been a similar explosion in the population of centenarians, with the result that survival to the age of 100 is no longer the newsworthy feat that it was only a few decades ago. U.S. Census projections already forecast dramatic increases in the number of centenarians in the next 50 years: 4 million in 2050, compared to 37,000 in 1990.

Although Census Bureau calculations project an increase in average lifespan of only eight years by the year 2050,[2] some experts believe that the human lifespan should not begin to encounter any theoretical natural limits before 120 years.[3] With continuing advances in molecular medicine and a growing understanding of the aging process, that limit could rise to 130 years or more.

AGING AS A TREATABLE CONDITION

Aging is typically accompanied by increased vulnerability to illness, but it also exhibits physical manifestations that are not connected to any particular disease process. Characteristic signs include diminished appetite, general muscle weakness and unsteadiness of gait, thinning of the skin, and decreases in lung and kidney function. Together these contribute to the overall frailty of old age and are indicators of a process that, even in the absence of an identifiable disease, constitutes a slow withering away. This elusive process will be the object of intense scrutiny in the decades ahead.

Much insight has been derived from the study of Werner's syndrome, a rare genetic disorder in which the normal aging clock is dramatically and disastrously accelerated. The disease results in the uncanny phenomenon of patients in their teens and twenties with gray hair, cataracts, atrophied muscles, and loss of bone mass that would be normal only for the very old. Skin biopsies show tissue structures very similar to those of the aged, and cells demonstrate a sharply diminished ability to replicate. The premature aging and early death of Werner's patients, once an enigma, now appears to be the result of a defect in a gene that induces production of an abnormal "helicase" protein. This protein interferes with the body's normal process of DNA repair, the failure of which now appears to be a key feature of premature aging. Defective helicase also appears to exert other widespread damage, giving rise to cancer, early heart disease, and rare skin diseases. Identification of the roles of helicase and DNA repair in the bizarrely accelerated aging process of Werner's syndrome has obvious implications for our understanding of normal aging.[4]

On the other side of the coin, researchers studying roundworms have demonstrated that four genes, when mutated, cause the roundworm to live almost five times longer than its natural life expectancy—nearly two months rather than the normal nine days. Worms with this "long life" mutation have a lower metabolic rate, eat and move more languidly, and generally exhibit a more placid pace of life. (Is there a lesson for humans here?) These findings have been interpreted to suggest that the "rate of living" is a key determinant of degeneration and death. The slower life, it is thought, may reduce the rate of production of toxic oxidative by-products of metabolism (free radicals) that damage DNA, or it may allow the damage to be repaired more readily. All of these explanations are speculative, but the fact that a genetic alteration can extend life seems clear.[5]

The first attempt to slow down the wear and tear of aging has focused on helping the body eliminate the highly reactive free radical molecules that inflict damage on DNA, cell proteins, and other critical biological substances. The body has its own defenses against free radicals, including naturally occurring antioxidants. To boost these defenses, a variety of supplementary antioxidants, including vitamins C and E, beta-carotene, and selenium, have been suggested as therapies. Antioxidant administration in animals modestly extends life, but there is no evidence that current anti-oxidant supplements have a similar effect in humans. Antioxidant therapy is a landmark, however, in the acceptance of aging as a treatable condition.

An important biological phenomenon, programmed cell death, opens another avenue of exploration. Normal cells grown in a test tube can divide no more than about 50 times before a "cell death" program is activated. The program is apparently mediated by the loss of telomeres from the caps at the ends of each chromosome. As I noted in the discussion of cancer's molecular origins, these caps protect the genes in the chromosome from injury and allow cell division to proceed normally. As cells divide, the telomere cap shortens at each replication, and when the cap shortens sufficiently, a signal blocks further multiplication of the cell, and it dies. Can this loss of telomeres be prevented and the cells thereby kept from aging and dying? The most promising approach to preserving telomeres focuses on the naturally occurring enzyme telomerase, which has the capacity to synthesize new caps on chromosomes. Techniques for stimulating telomerase activity may therefore maintain the integrity of telomere caps, prolong the life of cells, and extend the life of the organism, so long as uncontrolled, cancerous cell growth can be avoided.[6]

Because many other factors are involved in aging, it is unlikely that telomerase activation alone will be the magic answer to senescence. But taken together with the discoveries concerning the effects of free radicals and of the helicase protein's role in Werner's disease, the findings suggest that we are entering a new era in the understanding of aging. Whether this work will lead to major changes in our clinical understanding and control of aging and its diseases is still not clear. But conceivably by 2050, aging may in fact prove to be simply another disease to be treated.

THE SOCIAL CONSEQUENCES OF AN EXTENDED LIFESPAN

Every change in human society, no matter how seemingly beneficial, brings with it the potential for new problems, and the continuing conquest of human disease is no exception. Concern over cancer, heart disease, and other illnesses, and over the costs of associated health care may be alleviated only to be replaced by the threat of a population explosion in which the extraordinarily long-lived elderly become an overwhelming social problem.

Overpopulation as a threat to mankind is, of course, not a new issue. Around 1800 Thomas Malthus argued that because of the natural exponential growth of populations, a stable population could be maintained only through wars, famine, and plague or, less plausibly, voluntary "moral restraint." But overpopulation first surfaced as a major policy concern around 1960, evidenced by publication of an influential report by the Club of Rome dealing with the limits to population growth and Paul Ehrlich's widely read book The Population Bomb. These and other similar commentaries at that time regarded high birth rates as the root of the population crisis.

But as long ago as the 1950s—just about the time that the DNA double helix was discovered—science fiction writers began to envision the time when overpopulation would occur as the result of the life-extending miracles of modern medicine. In his 1953 short story "Tomorrow and Tomorrow and Tomorrow," Kurt Vonnegut Jr. presents a humorous but believable vision of a society paralyzed by the burden of an older generation that has worn out its welcome, as typified by this exchange:

"Sometimes I get so mad, I feel like just up and diluting his anti-gerasone," said Em.

"That'd be against Nature, Em," said Lou, "it'd be murder. Besides, if he caught us tinkering with his anti-gerasone, not only would he disinherit us, he'd bust my neck. Just because he's one hundred and seventy-two doesn't mean Gramps isn't strong as a bull."

"Against Nature," said Em. "Who knows what Nature's like anymore? Ohhhh—I don't guess I could ever bring myself to dilute his anti-gerasone or anything like that, but, gosh, Lou, a body can't help thinking Gramps is never going to leave if somebody doesn't help him along a little. Golly—we're so crowded a person can hardly turn around, and Verna's dying for a baby, and Melissa's gone thirty years without one." She stamped her feet. "I get so sick of seeing his wrinkled old face, watching him take the only private room and the best chair and the best food, and getting to pick out what to watch on TV, and running everybody's life by changing his will all the time."[7]

The widely discussed film *Soylent Green*, made in 1973 and based on a 1966 short story by Harry Harrison, depicts a macabre program of mass extermination as a way to deal with the overpopulation caused by medical progress. And many other science fiction works of the 1960s and '70s depict organized euthanasia as a solution to the problem, the victims being chosen by a variety of creative methods ranging from random lottery to selective culling of the old, infirm, or politically suspect.[8] Some of the most chilling scenarios involve the use of the medical profession to assist in the killing. One story, for instance, imagines the replacement of ten percent of the supplies of a vaccine with a placebo in order to permit a randomly-selected portion of the population to be eliminated through infectious disease. Only slightly less grotesque are the short stories that imagine enforced restrictions on reproduction as a way out of the overpopulation dilemma. Jose Farmer's 1985 novel *Dayworld* offers yet another approach to the problem: he envisions a world in which every person is conscious for only one day out of seven and spends the rest of the time stacked in a storage facility (a tactic that contemporary office workers might argue has already been enacted).[9]

These imaginative speculations may offer few practical lessons, but they do show that thoughtful people have begun to consider medical advancement as a two-edged sword, not only because of the economic consequences discussed throughout this book but also because it threatens to distort the natural cycle of birth, aging, and death. Although restrictions on reproductive freedom or a mandated approach to euthanasia may today seem unthinkable, in another fifty years the severity of the population problem may be such that all conceivable solutions will be on the table.

Perhaps the most likely near-term response to the problem is that government policymakers could direct medical research funding toward work that increases quality of life rather than length of life. Research funding could be curtailed for some of the genetic interventions discussed earlier in favor of attention to such problems as loss of hearing and eyesight, degenerative skin diseases, and other indignities of old age. Even this relatively benign strategy for slowing the rise in life expectancy is likely to encounter stiff opposition, and any deliberate stifling of scientific progress is, of course, a cause for concern. We can only hope that as the contours of the dilemma become clearer in the decades ahead, creative minds will forge solutions that can avoid the world of Vonnegut's imagining. It may also be that life-extending medical progress will eventually plateau for purely scientific reasons, and that the vision of a society dominated by 130-year-olds will never materialize. But the medical successes of recent decades provide ample reason for us to plan for the possibility of a world in which disease and death are pushed ever farther into the second century of life.

Epilogue

Where does all this leave us as we try to sort out the challenges that face us at the beginning of a new century? We are enticed by visions of triumph over disease but disturbed by the near-term prospect of denying useful care to some patients. We are enthralled by the breakthrough achievements of researchers and clinicians but concerned that no clear code of behavior governs physicians and other health care providers. We look forward to a time when genetic targeting of disease may once again make health care affordable for all but confront a health insurance system that creates a hierarchy of access to quality care. We attempt to squeeze every drop of waste and inefficiency from the health-care system but witness an apparently inexorable climb in costs. The dichotomy of medicine's immense potential and the constraints that limit its realization has never been sharper.

As government budgets become increasingly ransomed to health care costs and as employers are forced to divert more and more of workers' wages to health insurance premiums, the need for effective solutions to these dilemmas is reaching a critical juncture. One policy approach would be to cut back on the fuel for the medical R&D machine by reducing government funds for biomedical research. But the American people have come to take medical progress for granted, and they continue to put medical research near the top of the list of worthwhile government programs. The only near-term, equitable alternative to comprehensive cuts in research programs is to restrict the availability of expensive therapies to those patients who are likely to derive the most significant benefits from them and to deny access to those patients who are likely to derive only a marginal benefit. Americans resist the idea of rationing, but HMOs and other managed care plans are already tacitly rationing medical services. This trend is likely to continue, and there will be increasing pressure from health care consumers to make these decisions explicit and bring them under regulatory and legal control.

Explicit forms of rationing, however, may prove to be so much at odds with the prevailing ethos of health care entitlement that they will be accepted only on a very gradual and limited basis. The attractiveness of current managed care models is that although they limit health care dollars, they make no single practitioner or government agency answerable for specific actions that limit access to care. Managed care providers can be expected to defend this comfortably nebulous status quo, and patients themselves may feel they have a better chance of getting the care they want in a system of pervasive but discretionary rationing as opposed to one in which specific rationing strategies are mandated for all patients. Such an amorphous system may be as politically inevitable as it is logically indefensible.

One of the most fascinating and critical developments in the coming years will be the evolving role of government in regulating managed care. On the one hand, government agencies will continue to encourage managed care models as a way to hold down state and federal insurance expenditures and respond to the needs of employers and other payers. On the other hand, politicians are already finding themselves compelled to regulate quality of care in the managed care industry in response to the complaints of increasingly vociferous patient advocacy groups. The resulting regulations, such as bans on mandated short hospital stays for childbirth, assuage patients but blunt the cost-saving potential of managed care. The stage is thus set for a powerful and increasingly consolidated managed care industry doing more or less constant battle with a government caught between its competing goals of cost containment and consumer protection.

Similarly, the idea of an all-inclusive, government-run health care system may now be political poison, but there is nevertheless growing support in Congress for expanding health care coverage for infants and children. Provision for other previously uninsured patients in the health care system could follow, but these goals are probably unattainable without greatly increased government involvement in the health care system. Furthermore, the trend toward consolidation of managed care and provider organizations into larger and larger for-profit corporations raises significant antitrust issues that can be addressed only through increasing government intervention. The Clinton national health insurance plan is now viewed as a case study in political miscalculation, but many features of the plan may well reappear in the decades ahead.

The next 25 years will be especially challenging and possibly divisive ones, but it is important that we not lose sight of the utopian visions that are emerging. The possibility of mastery over a broad range of illnesses is no longer the sole property of philosophers and science fiction authors. Our challenge will be to tackle the ethical and social issues that accompany medical progress with the same rigor that we apply to the scientific challenges themselves. Above all we must ensure that in the sacrifices required to realize our visions, especially in the critical area of health care rationing, we do not compromise fairness and equity, without which the conquest of disease would be a hollow victory.

Notes

1 Quoted in Rolleston HD. *Some medical aspects of old age.* London: Macmillan, 1922, 7.
2 Quoted in Dubos R. *The dreams of reason: Science and utopias.* New York: Columbia University Press, 1961, 64–56.
3 Americans share Nobel for cell signal finding. *New York Times* 11 October 1994:B5, B6.

1 Drew EB. The health syndicate. *Atlantic Monthly* 1967;220(6):75–82.
2 Strickland SP. *Politics, science, and dread disease.* Cambridge, Mass.: Harvard University Press, 1972; National Institutes of Health Web page: www.nih.gov/news/budget.
3 Calculation based on data from the Health Care Financing Administration, Office of the Actuary, and on U.S. Bureau of Economic Analysis. *National income and product accounts of the United States: Volume 1, 1929–58.*
4 Rettig RA, Marks E. *The federal government and social planning for end-stage renal disease: past, present, and future.* Santa Monica, Calif.: Rand, 1983.
5 Rettig RA. *Origins of the medicare kidney disease entitlement: the social security amendments of 1972.* Washington, D.C.: National Academy of Sciences, Institute of Medicine, 1990.

6   Rettig RA. The policy debate on patient care financing for victims of end stage renal disease. *Law and Contemporary Problems* 1976; 40(4):196–230.

7   *United States renal data system 1996 annual report.* Bethesda: National Institutes of Health, 1996.

8   U.S. Department of Health, Education, and Welfare. *Health United States 1976–1977.* Hyattsville, MD.: DHEW, 1977; Tunis SR, Gelband H. Health care technology in the United States. *Health Policy* 1994;30:335–96.

9   Levit KR, Sensenig AL, Cowan CA, et al. National health expenditures, 1993. *Health care financing review* 1994;16(1):247–94.

10   Pierce EC. Anesthesiologists have led the way toward reform. *Washington Post* 19 November 1996; Health Section: 13, 15.

11   Calculation of health care inflation rate based on data from the Health Care Financing Administration, Office of the Actuary and from GDP implicit price deflator data from the Department of Commerce, Bureau of Economic Analysis. See also Newhouse JP, An iconoclastic view of health cost containment. *Health Affairs Supplement* 1993:152–71, and Schwartz WB, The inevitable failure of current cost-containment strategies: why they can provide only temporary relief. *Journal of the American Medical Association* 1987; 257(2):220–24.

12   Levit KR, Sensenig AL, Cowan CA, et al. National health expenditures, 1993. *Health Care Financing Review* 1994;16(1):247–94; and Health Care Financing Administration, Office of the Actuary: Data from the Office of National Health Statistics, 1997.

13   On foreign health spending, see Organization for Economic Cooperation and Development as cited in *Statistical abstract of the United States 1995*, Table 1369. On U.S. infant mortality, see U.S. Bureau of the Census, unpublished data as cited in the *Statistical abstract of the United States 1995*, Table 1363.

14   U.S. Bureau of the Census, unpublished data as cited in the *Statistical abstract of the United States 1995*, Table 1363.

15   U.S. Bureau of the Census. *Current population reports*, series P-60, no. 150 (1987) and earlier reports.

Chapter 2

1   Schwartz WB, Mendelson DN. Hospital cost containment in the 1980s: hard lessons learned and prospects for the 1990s. *New England Journal of Medicine* 1991;324:1037–42.

2   Calculations based on data from American Hospital Association, *Hospital Statistics 1995–96 Edition* (Chicago: AHA, 1995); see also Schwartz WB, Mendelson DN. Hospital cost containment in the 1980s: hard lessons learned and prospects for the 1990s. *New England Journal of Medicine* 1991; 324:1037–42.

3   *Managed health care: effect on employers' costs difficult to measure.* Washington, D.C.: United States General Accounting Office, 1993.

4   *Managed health care: effect on employers' costs difficult to measure.* Washington, D.C.: United States General Accounting Office, 1993.

5   Levit KR, Sensenig AL, Cowan CA et al. National health expenditures, 1993. *Health Care Financing Review* 1994;16(1):247–94.

6   Schwartz WB, Mendelson DN. Eliminating waste and inefficiency can do little to contain costs. *Health Affairs* 1994;13(1):224–38.

7   American Hospital Association, *Hospital statistics 1995–96 Edition.* Chicago: AHA, 1995.

8   Calculation based on American Hospital Association, *Hospital statistics 1995–96 Edition.* Chicago: AHA, 1995.

9   Schwartz WB, Mendelson DN. Eliminating waste and inefficiency can do little to contain costs. *Health Affairs* 1994;13(1):224–38.

10   American Hospital Association, *Hospital statistics 1995–96 Edition.* Chicago: AHA, 1995.

11   Audit of Medicare finds $23 billion in overpayments. *New York Times* 17 July 1997:A1.

12   U.S. contends billing fraud at Columbia was "systemic." *New York Times* 7 October 1997:C1, C4.

13   Sparrow MK. *Health care fraud control: the state of the art.* Cambridge: Harvard, 1995.

14   Aaron HJ, Schwartz WB. An ounce of prevention as costly as the cure. *Washington Post* 16 November 1995:A23

15   Aaron HJ, Schwartz WB. An ounce of prevention as costly as the cure. *Washington Post* 16 November 1995:A23.

16 Prager LO. Questions raised about impact of guidelines in Maine project. *American Medical News* 1996;39(21):1, 3.

17 *Acute pain management: operative or medical procedures and trauma.* Rockville, Md.: Agency for Health Care Policy and Research, 1992.

18 Calculations based on data from American Hospital Association, *Hospital statistics 1995–96 Edition.* Chicago: AHA, 1995.

19 Calculations based on data from American Hospital Association, *Hospital statistics 1996–97 Edition.* Chicago: AHA, 1996.

20 Aaron HJ. *Serious and unstable condition: financing America's health care.* Washington, D.C.: Brookings Institution, 1991.

21 Analysts expect health premiums to rise sharply. *New York Times* 19 October 1997:1, 14.

22 Government worker premiums to rise 8.5%. *Hospitals and Health Networks* 1997; 71(20):83.

23 Schwartz WB, Mendelson DN. Eliminating waste and inefficiency can do little to contain costs. *Health Affairs* 1994;13(1):224–38.

24 Data from the Health Care Financing Administration are used throughout this discussion.

Chapter 3

1   Jensen GA, Morrisey MA, Gaffney S, Liston DK. The new dominance of managed care: insurance trends in the 1990s. *Health Affairs* 1997;16(1): 125–36.

2   Rosenthal E. Patients with rare illnesses fight new H.M.O.'s to get treatment. *New York Times* 15 July 1996:A1, B4.

3   Maker of cancer drugs to oversee prescriptions at 11 cancer clinics. *New York Times* 15 April 1997:A1, D4.

4   *National survey of employer-sponsored health plans/1995.* New York: Foster Higgins, 1995.

5   Association of American Medical Colleges. *Facts: applicants, matriculants and graduates, 1988–1994.* AAMC, 1994.

6   Mitka M. Market-driven match: most U.S. grads choose primary care. *American Medical News* 1996;39(14):1,7; Schroeder SA. The latest forecast: managed care collides with physician supply. *Journal of the American Medical Association* 1994;272(3):239–40.

7   A.M.A. and colleges assert there is a surfeit of doctors. *New York Times* 1 March 1997:7.

8   Physician Payment Review Commission. Annual report to Congress. Washington, D.C., 1995.

9   Congress urged to limit foreign medical residents in U.S. *Chronicle of Higher Education* 7 March 1997.

10   American Medical Association. *Physician characteristics and distribution in the U.S., 1995–96 Edition.* Chicago: AMA, 1996.

11   Schwartz WB, Mendelson DN. Physicians who have lost their malpractice insurance. *Journal of the American Medical Association* 1989;262(10): 1335–41.

12   A.M.A. and colleges assert there is a surfeit of doctors. *New York Times* 1 March 1997:7.

13   U.S. to pay hospitals to train fewer doctors to reduce glut. *New York Times* 25 August 1997:A12, A16.

Chapter 4

1   Raichle ME. Visualizing the mind. *Scientific American* 1994;270(4):58–63.

2   Satava RM. Emerging medical applications of virtual reality: a surgeon's perspective. *Artificial Intelligence in Medicine* 1996;6(4):281–88.

3   Schoenenberger AW, Bauerfeind P, Krestin GP, et al. Virtual colonoscopy with magnetic resonance imaging: in vitro evaluation of a new concept. *Gastroenterology* 1997;112(6):1863–70.

4   Satava RM. Virtual reality and telepresence for military medicine. *Computers in Biology and Medicine* 1995;25(2);229–36.

5   Schwartz WB, Patil RS, Szolovitz P. Artificial intelligence in medicine: where do we stand? *New England Journal of Medicine* 1987;316:685–88.

6   Baxt WG. Use of an artificial neural network for the diagnosis of myocardial infarction. *Annals of Internal Medicine* 1991;115(11):843–48.

7   Baxt WG, Skora J. Prospective validation of artificial neural network trained to identify acute myocardial infarction. *Lancet* 1996;347(8993): 12–15.

8   Pivotal trial of artificial skin advances tissue engineering industry. *Genetic Engineering News* 15 January 1996:25.

9   Rubel EW, Stone JS. Stimulating hair cell regeneration: on a wing and a prayer. *Nature Medicine* 1996;2(10):1082–83.

10 Skin grown in the lab offers hope for burns and unhealable wounds. *New York Times* 28 June 1995:B6. Swedish team treats knee injuries with laboratory-grown cartilage cells. *Genetic Engineering News* 15 October 1994:3.

11 Langer R and Vacanti JP. Artificial organs. *Scientific American.* September 1995:130–33.

12 Preston J. Trenton votes to put strict limits on use of gene tests by insurers. *New York Times* 18 June 1996:A1, B6.

13 Preston J. Trenton votes to put strict limits on use of gene tests by insurers. *New York Times* 18 June 1996:A1, B6.

14 Wilmut I, Schnieke AE, McWhir J, Kind AJ, Campbell KH. Viable offspring derived from fetal and adult mammalian cells. *Nature* 1997; 385(6619):810–13.

15 With cloning success, ethics issues intensify. *Los Angeles Times* 24 February 1997: A1, A14.

Chapter 5

1   Aaron HJ and Schwartz WB. *The painful prescription: rationing hospital care.* Washington, D.C.: Brookings Institution, 1984.

2   Organization for Economic Cooperation and Development, Paris, France, cited in *Statistical abstract of the United States,* 1995: Table 1369.

3   Maynard A, Bloor K. Introducing a market to the United Kingdom's National Health Service. *New England Journal of Medicine* 1996:334(9): 604–7; Light D, May A. *Britain's health system: from welfare state to managed markets.* New York: Faulkner & Gray, 1993.

4   Aaron HJ, Schwartz WB. *The painful prescription: rationing hospital care.* Washington, D.C.: Brookings Institution, 1984, 102.

5   Aaron HJ, Schwartz WB. *The painful prescription: rationing hospital care.* Washington, D.C.: Brookings Institution, 1984, 102.

6   Dean M. British health rationing becomes explicit. *Lancet* 1995;346: 1415.

7   All quotations in this discussion taken from Rising costs threaten generous benefits in Europe. *New York Times* 6 August 1996: A1, A4.

8   Woolhandler S, Himmelstein DU, Lewontin JP. Administrative costs in U.S. hospitals. *New England Journal of Medicine* 1993;329(6): 400–403.

9   Danzon PM. Hidden overhead costs: is Canada's system really less expensive? *Health Affairs* 1992; 11(1):21–43.

10   McKendry RJR, Wells GA, Dale P, et al. Factors influencing the emigration of physicians from Canada to the United States. *Canadian Medical Association Journal* 1996;154(2):171–81.

Chapter 6

1   Schwartz WB, Mendelson DN. Why managed care cannot contain hospital costs—without rationing. *Health Affairs* 1992;11(2):100–107.

2   Luft HS. *Health maintenance organizations: dimensions of performance.* New York: Wiley, 1981.

3   Luft HS. Trends in medical care costs. *Medical Care* 1980; 18:1–16; Newhouse JP, Schwartz WB, Williams AP, Witsberger C. Are fee-for-service costs increasing faster than HMO costs? *Medical Care* 1994;23:960–66.

4   Schwartz WB. A serious threat to HMO's health. *Wall Street Journal* July 7, 1988:22.

5   New York state faults Medicaid H.M.O.'s on care. *New York Times* 17 November 1995:A19.

6   Cost-cutting firms monitor couch time as therapists fret. *Wall Street Journal* 13 July 1995:A1, A9.

7   Kaiser/Harvard National Survey of Americans' Views on Managed Care. 1997. Full survey results and commentary available at the Kaiser Family Foundation Web site: www.kff.org.

8   Kassirer JP. Managing managed care's tarnished image. *New England Journal of Medicine* 1997;337(5):338–39.

9   Jollis JG, DeLong ER, Peterson ED, et al. Outcome of acute myocardial infarction according to the specialty of the admitting physician. *New England Journal of Medicine* 1996;335(25):1880–87; Selby JV, Fireman BH, Lundstrom RJ, et al. Variation among hospitals in coronary-angiography practices and outcomes after myocardinal infarction in a large health maintenance organization. *New England Journal of Medicine* 1996;335:1888–96.

10   Schwartz KB. A patient's story. *Boston Globe Magazine* 7 November 1994: 1, 15, 17–20, 23–37.

11   Calculation based on Waldo DR. Health expenditures by age group, 1977 and 1987. *Health care financing review* (Summer 1989): 114.

12   Emmanuel EJ. Cost savings at the end of life: what do the data show? *Journal of the American Medical Association* 1996;275(24):1907–14.

Chapter 7

1   Schwartz WB. The inevitable failure of current cost-containment strategies: why they can provide only temporary relief. *Journal of the American Medical Association* 1987; 257(2):220–24; Aaron HJ. *Serious and unstable condition: financing America's health care.* Washington, D.C.: Brookings, 1991; Newhouse JP. An iconoclastic view of health cost containment. *Health Affairs Supplement* 1993;152–71.

Chapter 8

1   Mariner WK. Patients' rights after health care reform: who decides what is medically necessary? *American Journal of Public Health* 1994;84(9): 1515–20.

2   Hall MA and Anderson GF. Health insurers' assessment of medical necessity. *University of Pennsylvania Law Review* 1992;140:1637–712.

3   Anderson GF. The courts and health policy: strengths and limitations. *Health Affairs* 1992;11(4):95–110.

4   Hall MA and Anderson GF. Health insurers' assessment of medical necessity. *University of Pennsylvania Law Review* 1992;140:1637–712.

5   *Wickline v State of California.* 228 Ca. Rptr. 661.

6   Stone AA. Law's influence on medicine and medical ethics. *New England Journal of Medicine* 1985;312(5):309–12; Schuck PH. Malpractice liability and the rationing of care. *Texas Law Review* 1981;59:1421–27; Havighurst CC. Prospective self-denial: can consumers contract today to accept health care rationing tomorrow? *University of Pennsylvania Law Review* 1992;140 (5): 1755–808.

7   Anderson GF. The courts and health policy: strengths and limitations. *Health Affairs* 1992;11(4):95–110. Hall MA, Anderson GF. Health insurers' assessment of medical necessity. *University of Pennsylvania Law Review* 1992;

140:1637–712. Bergthold LA, Sage WM. Medical necessity, experimental treatment and coverage determinations: lessons from national health reform. Washington, DC: National Institute for Health Care Management, 1994.

8   Barnett v Kaiser Foundation Health Plan, Inc. 1994 WL 400819 (9th Cir.(Cal.)).

9   Schwartz WB, Komesar NK. Doctors, damages, and deterrence: an economic view of medical malpractice. New England Journal of Medicine 1978; 298:1282–89.

10 Prosser WL. Handbook of the Law of Torts. 4th ed. St. Paul, Minnesota: West Publishing, 1971, 145.

11 United States v Carroll Towing Co. 159 Fed. Rptr. 2d 169 (1947).

12 Schwartz WB, Komesar NK. Doctors, damages and deterrence: an economic view of medical malpractice. New England Journal of Medicine 1978; 298:1283.

13 Patients, doctors, and lawyers: medical injury, malpractice litigation, and patient compensation in New York. Harvard Medical Practice Study. 1990.

14 Fox DM and Schaffer DC. Semi-preemption in ERISA: legislative process and health policy. American Journal of Tax Policy 1988;7(1):48–69; Conison J. ERISA and the language of preemption. Washington University Law Quarterly 1994;72(2):619–69; McDonough RS. ERISA preemption of state-mandated provider laws. Duke Law Journal 1985:1194–1216.

15 1995 New York State Conference of Blue Cross Blue Shield Plans v Travelers Insurance Co. 115 SAT 1671.

16 Mariner WK. Liability for managed care decisions: the Employee Retirement Income Security Act (ERISA) and the uneven playing field. American Journal of Public Health 1996;86(6):863–69.

17 Spurred by public's complaints, Congress offers managed-care cures. Los Angeles Times 22 October 1997:A6.

Chapter 9

1   Marshall E. Gene therapy's growing pains. Science 1995;269(5227): 1050–55; Marshall E. Less hype, more biology needed for gene therapy. Science 1995;270:1751.

2   Gene therapy gives blood a path around leg blockages, researchers

say. *New York Times* 10 November 1997:A14; Roush W. Counterfeit chromosomes for humans. *Science* 1997;276(5309):38–39; Rosenfeld MA. Human artificial chromosomes get real. *Nature Genetics* 1997; 15(4):333–35.

3   Isis pharmaceuticals demonstrates efficacy in Crohn's disease with its antisense drug. *Genetic Engineering News* 1 March 1997;17(5):1, 34.

4   Marx J. Mutant enzyme provides new insights into the cause of ALS. *Science* 1996;271:446–47.

5   Davies SW, Turmaine M, Cozens BA, et al. Formation of neuronal intranuclear inclusions underlies the neurological dysfunction in mice transgenic for the HD mutation. *Cell* 1997;30(3):537–48.

6   Welsh MJ, Smith AE. Cystic fibrosis. *Scientific American* December 1995: 52–59.

7   Goldman MJ, Anderson GM, Stolzenberg ED, et al. Human B-defensin-1 is a salt-sensitive antibiotic in lung that is inactivated in cystic fibrosis. *Cell* 1997;88(4):553–60.

8   Meitinger T. Widening the view. *Nature Genetics* 1997;15(3):224–25; Vogel G. Glaucoma gene provides light at the end of the tunnel. *Science* 1997;275(5300):621.

9   Randall T. First gene therapy for inherited hypercholesterolemia a partial success. *Journal of the American Medical Association* 1993;269(7):837–38; Grossman M, Rader DJ, Muller DW, et al. A pilot study of ex vivo gene therapy for homozygous familial hypercholesterolaemia. *Nature Medicine* 1995;1(11):1148–54.

10 Soonpaa MH, Koh GY, et al. Formation of nascent intercalated disks between grafted fetal cardiomyocytes and host myocardium. *Science* 1994; 264(5155):98–101; Soonpaa MH, Daud AI, Koh GY, et al. Potential approaches for myocardial regeneration. *Annals of the New York Academy of Sciences* 1995;752:446–54.

11 Murry CE, Kay MA, Bartosek T, et al. Muscle differentiation during repair of myocardial necrosis in rats via gene transfer with MyoD. *Journal of Clinical Investigation* 1996;98(10):2209–17.

12 Isner JM, Walsh K, Symes J, et al. Arterial gene transfer for therapeutic angiogenesis in patients with peripheral artery disease. *Human Gene Therapy* 1996;7 (8):959–88; Isner JM, Pieczek A, et al. Clinical evidence of an-

giogenesis after arterial gene transfer of phVEGF165 in patient with ischemic limb. *Lancet* 1996;348(9024):370–74; Isner JM. The role of angiogenic cytokines in cardiovascular disease. *Clinical Immunology and Immunopathology* 1996;80(3 Pt 2):S82–91.

13 Takeshita S, Tsurumi T, et al. Gene transfer of naked DNA encoding for three isoforms of vascular endothelial growth factor stimulates collateral development in vivo. *Laboratory Investigation* 1996; 75(4):487–501.

14 Gene therapy gives blood a path around leg blockages, researchers say. *New York Times* 10 November 1997:A14.

15 The National Institute of Neurological Disorders and Stroke rt-PA Stroke Study Group. Tissue plasminogen activator for acute ischemic stroke. *New England Journal of Medicine* 1995;333(24):1581–87.

16 Barinaga M. Finding new drugs to treat stroke. *Science* 1996; 272(5262):664–66.

17 Castillo J, Davalos A, Noya M. Progression of ischaemic stroke and excitotoxic aminoacids. *Lancet* 1997;349(9045):79–83; Dorlando KJ, Sandage BW Jr. Citicoline (CDP-choline): mechanisms of action and effects in ischemic brain injury. *Neurological Research* 1995;17(4):281–84; Barinaga M. Finding new drugs to treat stroke. *Science* 1996;272(5262):664–66.

18 von-Herrath MG, Oldstone MB. Virus-induced autoimmune disease. *Current Opinion in Immunology* 1996;8(6):878–85; Solimena M, De Camilli P. Coxsackie viruses and diabetes. *Nature Medicine* 1995; 1(1):25–26.

19 Gottlieb AB. Immunopathogenesis of psoriasis: the road from bench to bedside is a 2-way street. *Archives of Dermatology* 1997;133(6):781–82.

20 Weiner HL, Friedman A, et al. Oral tolerance: immunologic mechanisms and treatment of animal and human organ-specific autoimmune diseases by oral administration of autoantigens. *Annual Review of Immunology* 1994;12:809–37.

21 Weiner HL, Mackin GA, et al. Double-blind pilot trial of oral tolerization with myelin antigens in multiple sclerosis. *Science* 1993;259 (5099):1321–24.

22 Trentham DE, Dynesius-Trentham RA, et al. Effects of oral administration of type II collagen on rheumatoid arthritis. *Science* 1993; 261(5129):1727–30.

23 Weiner HL. Oral tolerance: immune mechanisms and treatment of autoimmune diseases. *Immunology Today* 1997;18(7):335–43.

24 Levy SB. Antimicrobial resistance: a global perspective. *Advances in Experimental Medicine and Biology* 1995;390:1–13.

25 Service RF. Antibiotics that resist resistance. *Science* 1995;270(5237): 724–27.

26 Onishi HR, Pelak BA, Gerckens LS, et al. Antibacterial agents that inhibit lipid A biosynthesis. *Science* 1996;274(5289):980–82.

Chapter 10

1 Calculations based on data from U.S. Bureau of the Census.

2 U.S. Bureau of the Census. Current population report, special studies: 65+ in the United States. Washington, D.C.: U.S. Government Printing Office, 1996; Social Security Administration, Office of the Actuary. Tables used in support of the 1995 *Trustees Report*, Alternative 2 Life Expectancy Series.

3 Finch CE, Pike MC. Maximum lifespan predictions from the Gompertz mortality model. *Journals of Gerontology, Series A, Biological and Medical Sciences* 1996;51(3):B183–94.

4 Pennisi E. Premature aging gene discovered. *Science* 1996;272(5259): 193–94.

5 Pennisi E. Worm genes imply a master clock. *Science* 1996; 272 (5264): 949–50.

6 Zakian VA. Telomeres: beginning to understand the end. *Science* 1995; 270(5242): 1601–7. Bodnar AG, Ouelette M, Frolkis M, et al. Extension of lifespan by introduction of telomerase into normal human cells. *Science* 1998; 279(5349): 349–52.

7 Vonnegut K. *Welcome to the monkey house.* New York: Delacorte, 1954.

8 "Overpopulation." *Encyclopedia of Science Fiction.* New York: St. Martin's, 1993, 901–2.

9 Farmer P. *Dayworld.* New York: Putnam, 1985.

Index

Designer: Steve Renick
Compositor: Binghamton Valley Composition, LLC
Text: 11.5/14.5 Johanna
Display: Franklin Gothic
Printer and Binder: Maple-Vail Book Manufacturing Group